Intermittent solution

The ultimate intermittent fasting guide for women to lose weight, reset metabolism and slow aging down in healthy way through the most efficient autophagy techniques

Susan Sanderson

Table of contents

Is intermittent fasting a good thing?

"Isn't breakfast the most substantial meal of the day?"

"Want to lose weight? Make sure you start your day with a healthy breakfast so that your metabolism starts working. Have your breakfast like kings, lunch as princes, and dinner as poor. "

"Want to lose more weight? Try to eat six little meals a day, so that your body works at maximum capacity all day long. "

Nowadays, we discover so much about the importance of starting the day early and breakfast for healthy living and weight control. There are even studies showing that those who consume the first meal early in the day lose more weight than those who consume the first meal late or skip meals. So when you start your day with breakfast, do you get healthier or lose more weight?

But with a skeptical approach can we ask the question: what if there is scientific research that shows that skipping breakfast is more effective for optimum efficiency, maximum muscle involvement and fat loss? If you are interesting in knowing the reply, then this is the book for you, so keep reading!

Intermittent fasting, i.e. intermittent fasting is not a diet; is a nutrition scheme. In other words, it is based on an informed decision to skip certain meals. Intermittent fasting based on consciously starving before a certain period after eating; it means choosing to eat your meals at certain times of the day (eating window) and not to eat at rest times (hunger window).

It is not easy to define the concept of intermittent fasting because there are many different ways to implement it correctly. Intermittent fasting is practiced in different concepts around the world. The usual common versions of intermittent fasting are:

1. Fasting every other day: fasting every other day, as the name suggests, is the name given to fasting every two days. Nothing is invincible on fasting days, that is, hunger windows, while on other days, an average of around 500 calories is eaten.

2. The warrior diet: the warrior diet (also called hunter or soldier diet) is a method imposing long periods of fasting and short periods of feasting when you can eat up to 90% of the whole amount of calories you have to eat during the day.

3. Fasting 16/8: when practicing 16/8, fasting is carried out 16 hours a day, and the eating window is fitted to the remaining 8 hours. Often, after dinner and eat the next day in the morning, breakfast is applied by skipping.

4. Ye-dur-ye: it is practiced 24 hours a day or two of the week by not eating anything. The rest of the week is free of nutrition.

5. 5: 2 diet: 5: 2 concept, 5 days a week while eating normal, the remaining two days of calorie intake is based on keeping between 500-600 calories.

- ➢ Regularly eating at a specific time interval: for example, eating only between the hour of 12:00 and 20:00 and skipping breakfast, some people who apply intermittent fasting can leave this interval for 6 hours or even 4 hours.

- ➢ Skipping two meals a day and not eating anything 24 hours a day: for example, having your dinner in your normal order and not eating anything until dinner the next day.

After the above explanations, the working logic of intermittent fasting may look like this; I'm i skipped meals and had less food in total. Therefore i will give more weight." This is partly true. By eliminating any meal, even if you eat more of your other meals, the total amount of calories you receive is reduced, and you are getting closer to losing weight. However, since not all calories have the same effect on the body, the hour you eat can change your body's response to calories.

How does intermittent fasting work?

When you perform intermittent fasting, your body works in different ways during times of hunger and satiety:

When you eat, your body processes and burns what you eat for several hours. Since the foods you eat give the body the materials it can burn to produce energy; the body uses what you consume as a source of energy, not the stored oil. This is especially true if you consume carbohydrates or sugars; because the body prefers to use sugar before any source.

In the hunger window, since the body does not have a recently consumed food source for use in energy production, it is directed to the fats stored in your body rather than sugar in the bloodstream or glycogen in the muscle and liver.

Burn fat = gain.

The fact that your body uses fat stored for energy also applies when you are doing sports while you are on hunger. Unable to find a ready source of glucose or glycogen, the body has to use its only energy source: fats stored in your cells.

So how does this work? The body responds to food by producing insulin. The more sensitive your body is to insulin, the more effective it is to use the nutrients you consume; therefore, it supports fat burning and muscle formation, on the other hand, when your body is most sensitive to insulin, the time after the hunger process.

The glycogen in your body (starch stored in your muscles/liver and used by the body as a fuel when it is needed) decreases during sleep, i.e. Hunger; during physical activity, it decreases even further and insulin sensitivity increases. So the food you consume right after the sport is stored most effectively: a large part as glycogen in your muscles, a part as energy for use in healing and resting, and a small amount as fat.

To compare this to a day when you don't use intermittent fasting: when your insulin sensitivity is at normal levels, carbohydrates and foods you consume to fill up your glycogen stores, the quantity of glucose in your blood reaches a sufficient level, and so most of what you eat is stored as fat. On the other hand, growth hormone secretion increases during fasting (both during sleep and at the end of hunger windows). Increased secretion of growth hormone, decreased insulin production and consequently increased insulin sensitivity while applying intermittent fasting, the body is ready for muscle development and fat loss.

To put it differently: intermittent fasting helps your body teach you to use the nutrients it consumes more efficiently. For many different physiological reasons, when applied correctly, intermittent fasting accelerates weight loss and muscle formation.

So why do all health books recommend eating 6 meals a day?

Here are the reasons why many nutrition and diet books recommend eating 6 meals a day:

1. When you eat, your body system has to burn extra calories to process the foods you consume. The theory works as follows; if you eat small meals all day long, your body regularly burns extra calories; your metabolism also works at the optimum capacity. However, this information is not correct. Whether you consume 2000 calories in a short time or broadcast all day; your body consumes the same amount of calories when processing these foods. Although the proposal to increase your metabolism rate by eating continuously seems to work in theory, it is unfortunately in practice in the classroom.

2. When you make your meals more frequent and smaller, your chances of over-eating your main meals are reduced. Although this information is partially correct; it is not necessary to eat six meals a day as long as you teach yourself portion control or control what you eat. On the other hand, you'll probably never feel full when you eat 6 small meals, and so your chances of turning your snacks to higher calorie options will increase.

In short, 6 meals a day does not work in practice, as it does not work at the point where you think it works.

Returning to the Stone Age; it was not possible for our ancestors to eat every 3 hours under the conditions they lived in that period. Our ancestors were only fed when they found food, and even in this case, their body had adapted to work all day.

A recent study published in the New York Times discussed the technique of verme losing weight by eating 6 meals a day". According to martin, one of the writers of lean gains, the most important implications of the research are as follows:

The suggestion of the study was to increase the frequency of eating by providing short-term hunger control and increasing the likelihood of dieting; furthermore, the predicted beneficial effects of increasing the frequency of eating were that it provided better intestinal peptides and thus greater weight loss. All three hypotheses were refuted under the conditions given in the research."

"it was accepted that increased food frequency would increase the likelihood of adhering to energy-restricting diets and, therefore, would facilitate weight loss with increased satiety. However, the results do not confirm this hypothesis. "

Remember what you eat is essential. Eating frequency; the amount you eat and the quality of the food you eat are not as important.

There are plenty of reasons why you should choose an intermittent fasting approach to schedule your meal plans every day. Before going into deeper details, you should start by considering the following simple reasons:

- not all calories taken affect the body in the same way; however, calorie restriction is one of the cornerstones of losing weight. When you practice intermittent fasting, whichever method you choose, you also make it easier to restrict the number of calories you take during the week. You are less likely to lose weight because you have received fewer calories than before.

- it makes your job easier, instead of feeding 6 small meals a day, you don't have to try to pack, pack and eat every 2-3 hours.

- it takes less time and money, you spend only 3-6 meals a day, while you spend less and less time and money for 3-6 meals a day, and you only spend 2 meals a day at intermittent fasting.

- it supports muscle gain and weight loss, intermittent fasting increases insulin sensitivity and growth hormone secretion, which are the cornerstones of muscle development.

Intermittent fasting is not a common side effect of intermittent fasting. Many people worry about intermittent fasting, the lack of energy that long-term hunger can cause, loss of focus and the feeling of hunger. The number of people, who think that energy will drop during the day, especially when skipping breakfast, isn't much less.

The first time you switch from eating throughout the day to intermittent fasting, your body may have a little strain. However, when you complete the transition process, your body will quickly adjust to the new order and work as well as the order you eat throughout the day. In a study examining participants during and at the end of a 48-hour fasting window, it was concluded that 2 cognitive performance, activity, sleep and psychological state were not adversely affected in 2-day calorie deficiency in healthy individuals".

"why do not i feel grumpy breakfast well?" she asks if you will; maybe you're eating habits are the reason for your crankiness. The body, used to eating at frequent intervals, will wait for you to eat every 3 hours, as learning. In other words, if you have breakfast every morning, your body will ask you to have breakfast every morning when it wakes up. We can say that this process has both physical and psychological origins.

If you re-train your body so that it does not expect to eat every day or throughout the day; with *ghrelin* hormone secretion, side effects will become less effective. Returning to the cave era, our ancestors were able to survive periods of abundance as well as periods of famine. Remember, long-term starvation requires 84 hours to modify glucose levels in the body negatively. So 16 or 24-hour hunger windows are not a time your body can't handle.

Important warning:

Intermittent fasting; it can be a challenging process for people with conditions such as blood sugar problems, hypoglycemia, diabetes. If you have any discomfort, you should consult your doctor or dietitian before starting intermittent fasting.

Can i develop muscle or gain weight during intermittent fasting?

Exactly! Steve Kamb applies intermittent fasting in the bodybuilding process; muscles while developing the body fat ratio in a small amount of the same amount of calories in this process while taking calories in the 8-hour windows underlines. As for the program:

> ➢ 11 am - heavy strength training during fasting

➢ 12 pm - consumption of ½ of daily calories immediately after sports

➢ 7 pm - consuming the remaining half of your daily calories as dinner

➢ 8 pm - 12 pm (next day): 16-hour fast

This program, which is also included in lean gains, is one of the most effective programs for intermittent fasting. According to another program by nate green, you can effectively develop muscle by holding 24-hour fasts on sundays every week. This method also challenges the "bulk & cut" method that is commonly used in bodybuilding. Compared to intermittent fasting and the classic bulk & cut method to develop muscle, when intermittent fasting:

- Your balance does not deteriorate: so you do not need to take 30 kilograms and give 25 to get 5kg muscle. So your body mass doesn't change much.

- You eat less, so your money stays in your pocket: instead of the weight you get, you need to consume as much muscle and fat as you need. Slowly, steadily, steadily and permanently, you gain muscle and strength.

- The concept of the holiday body does not interest you: we all want to look good, especially in the summer when the clothes are thinner and smaller. In a scenario where your muscles develop regularly, you don't have to worry about how you look at any stage of the process.

First, maybe in the fasting window for 15 hours instead of 16? Relax, because your body is a customizable machine and everything is not as black or white as you think. If your desire to change your diet stems from aesthetic concerns or athletic performance, of course, you should be more consistent and punctual; but in other cases, there is no point in stressing yourself.

Try to keep yourself busy. If you are sitting without doing anything and thinking about how hungry you are, the more the process will challenge you.

When applying intermittent fasting, there are a few tips that will increase your productivity and make your life easier:

- Start the hunger window immediately after a hearty meal. When you're satiated enough, the last thing you'll want to think about is eating.

- Be sure to match the 8 hours of the 16-hour fasting window to your sleep process.

- If you haven't eaten just before sleep, you'll have left behind the hunger window for about 8-12 hours. It can be operated in the last 4 hours, and you can also spend the last 1 hour.

- You can consume calorie-free drinks while in the hunger window; you can drink green tea to meet your caffeine need. If you require drinking water, black coffee or tea, do not push yourself too hard and listen to the sound of your body.

When changing your diet, do not forget to observe the changes in your body.

- If you are afraid that you will lose your muscle mass, follow your strength training program more closely.

- Be sure to measure your body fat regularly.

- Keep track of your calories; so you can closely observe how your body changes by consuming the same amount of food.

Different bodies can react differently to intermittent fasting; you will not know what your body reaction will be. Therefore, it is up to you to listen to your body and make the necessary changes during this process.

Intermittent fasting helps you lose weight while increasing your insulin sensitivity and growth hormone secretion; however, it is only one of the hundreds of factors that affect your body shape and health. Don't expect to get rid of your fat mass by just having breakfast. You should have healthy eating habits, consume more quality and healthy foods and try to get stronger. Intermittent fasting is just one of the factors that will contribute to your success.

Intermittent fasting has potential positive effects for people who want to lose weight or increase muscle mass. The male and female bodies react separately to the intermittent fasting, just as each can react differently to the same situation. So the most effective way to see if the fasting is right for you is to try.

Diet is everyone's dream: to lose weight while being able to eat anything you want for most of the week, paying attention to what you only eat for a day or two. Believe it or not: intermittent fasting is not only a slimming waist; it keeps your blood sugar level in balance, reduces inflammation and protects your heart health.

Although approaches to intermittent fasting are different, many studies highlight the benefits of intermittent fasting to your health.

From fasting for several hours every day to skipping meals two days a week, intermittent fasting is one of the easiest and immediate ways to maintain your health and achieve your weight goals.

Benefits of intermittent fasting

1. Supports weight loss.

One of the most notable advantages of intermittent fasting is that it accelerates fat burning and helps you get rid of excess. One of the reasons why many people are using intermittent fasting instead of traditional diets is that you ought not to keep track of what you eat and calories constantly.

Intermittent fasting provides the use of fat stores in your body as energy, accelerating fat burning and weight loss. When you eat, your body utilizes glucose as the main source of energy and stores the remaining nutrients as glycogen in your muscles and liver. When you don't provide a regular flow of glucose to your body, the body begins to break down glycogen to use it as a source of energy. As glycogen decreases, the body starts to look for alternative energy sources and turns to fat cells.

The similarity between the intermittent fasting and the ketogenic diet is that both force your body to use oil as an energy source, depriving you of carbohydrates.

In research conducted in 2015 focusing on the effects of fasting every other day, it was concluded that this fast reduced body weight by 7% and resulted in an average loss of 4kg of fat. Similar results were achieved with all-day fasting, which resulted in a 9% reduction in body weight. However, the effects of fasting on the muscles all day have not been adequately explained.

In another study focusing on 16/8 interval fasting, it was concluded that this method significantly reduces the body fat and maintains muscle mass and strength.

2. He's regulating his blood sugar

When you eat, carbohydrates are shredded into glucose and mixed into the blood. The hormone called insulin transports glucose from the bloodstream to the cells where it will be used as energy. However, if you have diabetes, insulin doesn't always work. In this case, blood sugar rises, causing problems such as fatigue, thirst and increased toilet need.

Some research on the subject, intermittent fasting regulates blood sugar, fast ups and downs have been concluded that prevent.

In one study, participants with diabetes fasted for an average of 16 hours daily for two weeks. At the end of two weeks, it was observed that the calorie intake decreased and there was a vital decrease in blood sugar levels in addition to weight loss.

In another study, fasting reduced blood sugar by 12% as well as insulin levels were reduced by about 53%. The result of the research is as follows: preventing insulin secretion makes insulin work more efficiently and makes your body more sensitive to the effects of insulin.

3. Protecting your heart

One of the most impressive aspects of intermittent fasting is its positive effects on heart health. Research shows that intermittent fasting protects your heart health by reducing the risk of certain heart diseases.

In one of the studies, it was concluded that intermittent fasting positively affected some of the factors supporting heart health. Intermittent fasting increases hdl cholesterol, which is known as good cholesterol and low cholesterol ldl and triglyceride rates.

In a study conducted in animals published in the journal of nutritional biochemistry, it was concluded that intermittent fasting increases adiponectin levels. Adiponectin is a hormone that performs a role in fat and sugar metabolism and protects against heart disease and heart attack.

In another study, it was observed that the chances of getting rid of a heart attack in rats fed with fasting by day increased by 66% compared to rats fed with a normal diet.

4. Ltiha planını reduces.

Inflammation, the body's typical response to disability. Chronic inflammation is a condition that can lead to chronic diseases. Some studies even suggest that chronic inflammation is associated with diseases such as heart attacks, diabetes, obesity and cancer.

5. It protects your brain.

In addition to protecting your heart health and keeping you away from diseases, some research has shown that intermittent fasting also helps maintain brain health.

A study of animals has shown that intermittent fasting improves cognitive functions and protects the brain against changes in memory and learning ability.

In another study on animals, it was concluded that intermittent fasting protects the brain of mice by affecting certain proteins involved in ageing the brain.

The anti-inflammatory impacts of intermittent fasting can also help slow the development of diseases such as Alzheimer's disease.

6. Reduces hunger

Leptin, also known as the fasting hormone, is a hormone produced by fat cells, signalling to stop eating. The level of leptin decreases when you are hungry, and the level of leptin increases when you start to saturate.

Since leptin is produced in fat cells, the body's leptin hormone is higher in overweight or obese people. However, high levels of circulating leptin can lead to leptin resistance and make it difficult to respond to signs of hunger.

In a study conducted with 80 participants, the researchers measured leptin levels during intermittent fasting and concluded that the amount of leptin was lower during fasting nights.

Low levels of leptin mean less leptin resistance, less hunger and more weight loss.

Warnings

Although intermittent fasting has many benefits to your health, intermittent fasting may not be the right diet for people with disorders such as gallstones, eating disorders, thyroid disorders.

For example, if your blood sugar is low, not eating all day can lower your blood sugar even further, causing tremors, heart palpitations and fatigue. If you have diabetes, you should ask your doctor before taking intermittent fasting.

If you have a history of eating disturbances, intermittent fasting may trigger past unhealthy eating symptoms. Intermittent fasting is not recommended for developmental children.

If you're sick, it's best not to take intermittent fasting so you can get the nutrients you regularly need to get better and feel better.

Pregnant women should also have a diet plan rich in vitamins and minerals, so intermittent fasting is not recommended. Since hormonal problems may occur in some women after intermittent fasting, it is beneficial to take a break from fasting on certain days of the week.

If you have gallbladder discomfort, fasting, gallbladder problems can lead to; it is recommended not to apply.

Finally, research has shown that intermittent fasting can affect thyroid hormone levels. If you have any thyroid problems, you should consult your doctor before intermittent fasting.

If you have an active life, there is no problem in doing sports while intermittent fasting? You can do sports on fasting days; however, do not force yourself too much and take care to drink plenty of water. If you have a hunger window that lasts longer than 72 hours, it is recommended that you limit your physical activity.

We are going to start this very important chapter with a simple question: does intermittent fasting have different effects on women and men? Although the scientific community is still not unanimous on this topic, it is highly likely that intermittent fasting affects men and women differently. For instance, paleo for women focuses on the negative effects of intermittent fasting for women. Another guide in mark's daily apple highlights the differences in the male and female body and explains how they are affected by intermittent fasting:

In one study, intermittent fasting increased insulin sensitivity in men, but not in women. Another study examined the effect of day-fasting on blood lipids. Triglycerides remained stable while HDL increased benign cholesterol in women; in men, HDL remained stable, while triglyceride rate decreased. Although the effect of intermittent fasting on blood lipids varies depending on gender, the results were found to be positive in both cases.

In another study, it was seen that body fat, weight, blood pressure, cholesterol, malignant LDL cholesterol and triglyceride rates decreased in obese women and obese men who applied intermittent fasting. It should be noted, however, that the participants were obese and that per menopausal women were excluded from the study and that these results may not be the same in weaker people or women who have not yet had menopause.

According to other studies, women who approached intermittent fasting lifestyle might be more likely to face changes to their menstrual cycles, and this might be due to the female body is usually more extremely sensitive to calorie restriction during the fertile life-cycle. Additionally, when calorie intake is low a small part of the brain called the hypothalamus usually reacts by chancing the secretion of important hormones that are supposed to control the menstruation; this is why the risk of irregular periods and infertility might increase. For these reasons, women should consider a different approach to intermittent fasting than the male one, with shorter fasting periods and fewer fasting days.

Luckily there are also lots of good effects women can benefit from approaching an intermittent fasting lifestyle, as it might reduce the risk of developing a number of chronic diseases. But we are going to deal with this very important topic in the next chapter.

General guidelines of IF for women

The following ones are, among others, the best and most famous types of intermittent fasting approaches for women:

- Crescendo Method: Fasting 12–16 hours for no more than two or three days per week. Fasting days should not be consecutive (for example, Monday, Wednesday and Friday or Saturday).

- Eat-stop-eat (also knows as "the 24-hour protocol"): A 24-hour full fast maximum twice per week). Usually everybody starts with 14–16 hour fasts and then gradually builds up to allow the body to became familiar with the hunger.

- The 5:2 Diet (also called "The Fast Diet"): it is based on a restriction of calories to 25% of the usual amount for no more than two days per week and then on eating "normally" the other five days. Again the two days should not be consecutive.

- The 16/8 Method (also called the "Leangains method"): Fasting for 16 hours a day and eating all calories needed in the eight-hour window. Again, much better to start with 14-hour fasts and then eventually increase to 16 hours.

Whichever you choose, never forget to eat well during the non-fasting periods. If you eat a large amount of unhealthy and fat foods during the non-fasting periods, you might largely reduce the positive effects of these approaches.

In short, intermittent fasting experiences of men and women can result in different; however, since we all have different bodies, there is nothing more natural than not having the same results as another. Therefore, to reach the most accurate information you can try to apply a program that suits you and see for yourself.

What effect does IF have on lipid levels? Do I have to count calories to lose weight? Can I have a cheat day?

The following answers to frequently asked questions are based mainly on human studies conducted by intermittent post expert Dr. Krista Waradi, associate professor of nutrition at the University of Illinois at Chicago. Varadi's main research interest lies in the metabolic health effects of alternating fasting and time-limited nutrition. She has published more than 10 clinical trials of periodic fasting interventions.

Does intermittent fasting contribute to longevity?

There are promising animal studies showing that dietary restriction, including calorie restriction and intermittent fasting, can, at least in some cases, extend healthy lifespan and delay aging of diseases in various species from yeast to mice and monkeys. The molecular mechanisms of these effects include the elimination or improvement of the function of aging cells or damaged cells that have been noted by the body and prevented from dividing. Intermittent fasting can lead to cell aging for cell recycling, which may ultimately improve the function of aging tissues.

However, it is very difficult to study the biomarkers of aging and aging cells in humans, especially because most people cannot or will not participate in lengthy intervention studies. Evidence from such human studies is rare, and areas of calorie restriction and IF are no exception.

Although PF (prolonged fasting) can theoretically improve tissue function, especially with regard to metabolic function and circadian rhythms, more research is needed on the effects of prolonged fasting on longevity and longevity.

Who can benefit most from intermittent fasting?

Intermittent fasting studies for people with type 2 diabetes or at risk for developing type 2 diabetes are still preliminary, and most studies in this area are still conducted on animal models. However, there are promising experimental results from Krista Varadi's lab related to improved glucose regulation over time. Recent studies have shown that IF may have a greater positive effect on insulin resistance than traditional calorie-restricted diets. Although more research is needed, diabetics and prediabetics can benefit most from IF.

All people with diabetes and prediabetic conditions should work with their healthcare provider before and during fasting in any form, as this intervention can change their medication needs and other symptoms.

What is the effect of intermittent fasting on lipid levels?

Time-limited feeding (12+ hours per day) and fasting alternations (500 calories every other day) lasting from six to eight weeks in human studies have been associated with lower cholesterol and triglycerides in adults. In periodic studies on an empty stomach involving several hundred subjects, Dr. Krista Varadi constantly observed a decrease in triglycerides by 20-30% for three months of regular fasting. She also observed a moderate decrease in LDL cholesterol, primarily among people with high cholesterol, an increase in total LDL particle size, and a moderate increase in HDL or "good" cholesterol. HDL levels can also increase with exercise and niacin supplementation.

How long can I wait until I feel the benefits of intermittent fasting?

Intermittent fasting can contribute to weight loss and can improve metabolic health over time, affecting nutrient transfer, circadian biology, and intestinal microbiome. These effects may take some time. Studies of weight loss in IF usually include interventions that last from three to six months. According to Dr.

Krista Varadi, most people participating in these studies need two to three months to lose 10 pounds. For people with diabetes or prediabetes who want to change their A1C or blood glucose levels, it usually takes at least three months for these levels to change significantly.

In a 2016 study on time-limited nutrition (all calories consumed in an 8-hour window every day) in combination with weight training in healthy men, study participants who followed a fasting program for eight weeks experienced a decrease in fat mass without significant changes in muscle mass. People who were starving also experienced a decrease in IGF-1 and an increase in adiponectin, a hormone that can be an insulin sensitizer in the liver and muscles and help improve glucose and fat metabolism.

It is important to find a diet or metabolic lifestyle that you can incorporate into your lifestyle in the long run, given the negative effects of the yo-yo diet on most people. According to Varadi, it will be useful for many people to continue a long post for a long time.

Do I need to count calories to lose weight?

One of the benefits of time-limited feeding (for example, according to a fasting schedule of 16: 8) is that many people experience a natural calorie restriction and weight loss without counting calories. In a study of time-limited feeding (fasting 16 hours a day), Dr. Krista Varadi found that most study participants naturally reduced their daily calorie intake by 300 calories on average and lost 3% of their body weight after a three-month period, even when instructed to eat normally.

Can I have a cheat day?

It is important to be flexible. Intermittent fasting is ideally a lifestyle, not a fancy diet. In Dr. Krista Varadi's research on alternative fasting, she tells people not to worry if they miss two or three days a year. Sometimes your fasting days may come during a holiday or during another family event, and it may be tenser to fasting than enjoying a piece of cake.

However, some people believe that "cheating" breaks their entire post. If you are the type of person who needs a large structure to succeed in healthy behavior, Varadi suggests not skipping his quick days for family events or other occasions. However, for most people, a casual cheating day will not significantly impede the progress of weight loss or metabolic health.

Should I worry about the possible negative consequences of skipping meals for my blood sugar?

A small study published in 2017 raised concerns about skipping breakfast (post-fasting), which creates an acute state of glucose intolerance in the muscles when you resume eating. There is some evidence, based on the natural daily cycles of insulin sensitivity, that it is better to skip lunch or start a long night fast early in the evening rather than skipping breakfast or starving until late in the evening. However, studies of acute fasting, which address the effects of 24 to 48 hours of fasting for people who may not be used to such periods of fasting, do not necessarily indicate what might happen to people who regularly practice fasting, Dr. Krista Varadi says.

Can I take any supplements to improve fasting?

Ketone ester supplements are available for mass consumption today that can increase blood ketones and help you achieve ketosis. For athletes, these supplements can help the body produce ketones, which can be useful as an energy source during strenuous workouts. However, if you are no longer following a ketogenic diet, these supplements give your body mixed signals in terms of whether it should primarily burn fats or sugars as fuel. These supplements may be ineffective or not necessarily safe for metabolic health in the long run, says Dr. Krista Varadi.

How long is it safe to fast?

Dr. Krista Varadi says fasting up to 24-36 hours is usually safe and well tolerated based on clinical studies. However, in terms of weight loss and maintaining regular 24-hour water fasting, it can be difficult to adhere to and accept it as a long-term medical practice. People with eating disorders should not practice IF unattended by a doctor. However, it has been found that alternative fasting during the day reduces feelings of depression and overeating in obese individuals, improving the perception of body image.

It is better for your metabolic health to adhere to a fasting regimen that you can easily follow over time, with the caveat that you should stop fasting and consult a doctor if you experience dizziness or significant discomfort, or if you risk losing weight, Intermittent fasting is not the only a way to improve your metabolic health; It is important to choose the composition and nutrition plan that are best for you in the long run.

There is limited research on the effects or safety of long-term periodic fasting for 3-5 days at a time.

Is intermittent fasting safe for me if I get cancer treatment?

You should consult your doctor or oncologist before practicing intermittent fasting during any type of cancer treatment. Intermittent fasting can be problematic during treatment, especially if you experience muscle exhaustion, poor nutrition, or other side effects from treatment. However, there is evidence from in vitro studies, animal studies, and early human clinical trials by Dr. Walter Longo of the USC Longevity Institute and colleagues that intermittent fasting or low-protein diets that mimic fasting can increase the sensitivity of cancer cells to the effects of chemotherapy, protecting healthy immune cells and other cells from side effects. The IGF-1R pathway (insulin-like growth factor receptor 1) appears to be involved in stem cells regeneration and rejuvenation of the immune system, but how this happens remains uncertain.

Studies of the benefits of IF for cancer patients undergoing chemotherapy based on the differential stress tolerance of cancer and non-cancerous cells are promising, but preliminary. Long-term fasting of the order of several days can have other side effects and should never be carried out without consulting a doctor, oncologist or other medical expert.

Can fasting adversely affect bone density?

There is no indication that intermittent fasting compromises bone health. In a study of postmenopausal women conducted in the laboratory of Dr. Krist Varadi, six months of alternating daytime fasting did not affect bone density according to DEXA scans.

Intermittent fasting: 3 basic mistakes of beginners

Here are the 3 most common mistakes that you need to avoid in order to succeed with periodic fasting.

Error 1: Fear of getting hungry

We all feel hungry. This is a part of life. Whether you practice periodic fasting or eat out of the boxes every 2 hours, you will experience a feeling of hunger from time to time.

Take for example, a year ago Tade was gaining weight and somehow he heard one phrase: "If you get hungry, it's too late." The bottom line was the concept that the body switches to a catabolic mode if you have a strong feeling of hunger.

Being hungry for several hours is quite normal. All your muscles will not disappear, as well as hundreds of those who practice periodic fasting and have fairly decent muscle mass.

His height is 188, weight, on average, 90 kg (or even more) all year round. He has been eating this way for many years, and thanks to this he has quality muscles. Usually once a week he goes hungry 24 hours, just to cleanse the body completely. And you know what? His muscles remain intact.

The results of your hard work will not disappear after several hours of fasting. The truth is that the digestive system can stop the digestive process at any time.

You cannot eat 16-18-20-22 and even 24 hours. Your body is a wonderful device that can and will adapt to various conditions. Short starvation, say, for 16 hours, will not cause significant muscle breakdown. A very large number of studies have already proven this.

You could even train hungry - without a pre-workout meal, it all depends on the day of the workout and the regimen. Sometimes you can even wait several hours after training to make my first meal.

Although after training your body might receive nutrients for an hour, this is not the point, but the fact that you try to make the feeling of hunger normal and natural. Do not be afraid of hunger. Think of your body as a fat burning stove. It burns fat until you stuff it with food. This can help cope with fear.

Error 2: Food, mainly prepared food

With any diet, periodic fasting or standard 6-8 meals per day, if you eat ready-made meals, you will not succeed in the long term. As the saying goes, you will not create a million dollar body using the dollar menu, and this is 100% true!

If you are having difficulty fighting fat reduction with intermittent fasting, you may make mistakes in your diet and or the amount of food you eat. You can't eat a couple of packets of cookies to interrupt a hunger strike and assume that everything is normal, because you have been starving for 16 hours and therefore you need to eat - this will not work.

If you follow any nutritional scheme, it is best to start with the basics. If it runs, swims, grows from the earth - eat it. If it is in a package, drop it. This works for almost any diet, and periodic fasting is no exception. I'm not saying that you need to follow the Paleo diet, but eating meat, vegetables, and healthy fats usually works.

Periodically, starving does not mean that you need to eat all shit all day, because you have little time to eat. You are what you eat - fill your body with good, high-quality, whole food and you will look like Rambo, fill it with candied quick-prepared garbage and will look like the majority of the population.

Error 3: Watching the clock, prepare for the feast

Suppose you start with the standard 16-8. Starve 16 hours, eat 8. If you sleep 8 hours a day, stop eating 4 hours before bedtime, and wait 4 hours before you eat, then in reality you have to go without food for only 8 hours. In fact, it is not so difficult to do without food, and to be honest, fasting is more of a psychological problem: learn to "put up with absence."

This is not philosophical, but there is a lot to learn about yourself: your vocation, your path and you can start with regular fasting, make it a principle of life. But many beginners become "watch slaves," who wait, plan, and think about eating again because they worry that they are "hungry." You are not hungry. Your body can go without food for many days.

The reality is that you are just bored or hung up on food. Try to look back at the last 16 hours and focus on your work, training, and your family. Your life will improve significantly if you start following periodic fasting. If you sit and look at the clock, wait and think about how to eat, of course, so go crazy for a short time, give in to the desire to give up.

At first it is difficult to switch from snacks every two hours from waking up to falling asleep to the lack of food hour after hour. Believe me, in about a week everything will be fine.

Just live your life.

Fill your time with what matters - it's more important than cooking, eating it every 120 minutes and washing dishes after it. You may unexpectedly find that with periodic fasting you become more productive compared to a regular diet.

This does not mean that you should certainly starve strictly 16 hours a day. If you do this for 14 hours on the first day, it will be great. Perhaps on the second day you can be hungry for all 16 hours. Perhaps you will be carried away by work or go on a trip with your family and will not eat 18 hours. the bottom line is that periodic fasting makes your life easier, more efficient, makes you a thin, bold, sexy person.

This does not mean dependence on hours or scheduled meals. Eat when needed. If you are hungry, pull a few hours before eating. The bottom line is to make fasting suitable for your lifestyle, and nothing else. Now you have an appropriate way to make such a decision, you have the opportunity not to follow the clock in fear that a catabolic process will begin, muscle loss.

This is not for everyone, but it may be for you. Try it; start little by little, progress in periodic fasting in a comfortable mode.

The idea of intermittent fasting arose after scientists were struck by the consequences of constant calorie restriction. A number of studies in many different animals have shown that limited nutrition during adulthood leads to a significant improvement in life and overall health.

The reasons for these improvements are not yet clear. Part of it seems to be that leaving without food gives the cells in the body the necessary break for maintenance and repair. But lack of food also causes cells to resort to alternative energy sources. Some of them, such as ketones - molecules created in the liver from processed fat - are useful.

The Fight against Diabetes in Mice and Men

Recent studies on the effects of intermittent fasting on diabetes have focused on intermittent fasting in particular. As a first step, researchers led by Walter Longo at the University of Southern California began by testing whether intermittent hunger can cure diabetes in mice. They used mutant mice that lack fatty hormone leptin to regulate food intake. These mice constantly overeat and become obese and diabetic in early adulthood.

Researchers found that after several months of periodic fasting an alternation of seven unlimited days of nutrition with four limited days diabetes was cured. This is an amazing result, but even more surprisingly, the reason for this.

The mice lost weight during periodic fasting, which of course helped. But that was not the whole story. Periodic fasting actually solved the problem directly at one of its sources: the pancreas.

Diabetes is a disease characterized by an excess of blood sugar, which actually means an excess of glucose in the blood. This is basically an insulin problem. Typically, insulin causes cells in the body to take glucose from the blood. But with diabetes, glucose remains in the blood because the cells no longer take it. This is partly because many cells lose their sensitivity to insulin, but also because the pancreas stops doing this.

It turns out that periodic fasting caused the pancreas to start producing insulin again. Days of limited nutrition gave the pancreas a rupture that allowed it to remove and recycle many of its cells. Then, when the mice started eating again, new cells appeared that were able to produce insulin.

Thus, the pancreas actually contracted within four limited days of eating, and within seven unlimited days of eating they cut. After several such cycles of constriction, recirculation and regrowth, the pancreas was almost as good as the new one.

The big question, of course, is whether periodic posts will turn out to be the same effects on people. The answer is not yet clear, but the initial guidelines from a recently published phase two clinical trial, again led by Longo, are promising.

In this study, 100 people went through a 30-day cycle of periodic fasting, each with 25 days of unlimited nutrition and five days of limited nutrition. After only three cycles, those subjects who started the study with high blood sugar saw major improvements. And, importantly, not one of the subjects experienced any harmful effects.

Thus, evidence in support of intermittent fasting continues to grow. Does this mean that we should all do this? Not necessary.

Intermittent fasting seems most beneficial to those who are already overweight and unhealthy. Although it also appears to have some advantages for thin and healthy laboratory animals, it is not yet clears whether this is the same for humans.

Conversation Soon, a much larger phase of three trials of intermittent fasting in humans will begin, which will clarify many things. The results will undoubtedly be very interesting.

Why is intermittent fasting and keto recommended?

Fasting on keto can be incredibly useful, especially if you have reached a plateau and do not see results only from a ketogenic diet. Although not required, keto-intermittent fasting can take the benefits of your diet to a new level and help optimize your health.

It is also believed that it accelerates ketosis, helping the body burn glycogen stores faster, which can help avoid the symptoms of keto flu and get faster results.

There are many keto and recurring success stories for the post, and there are several reasons why you might want to add them to your daily routine. In particular, keto fasting was associated with several advantages, including:

Improved heart health: According to a study published in PLOS One, Fasting is effective in raising cholesterol, which can potentially help reduce the risk of heart disease.

Increased weight loss: Studies show that fasting can reduce body weight and body fat, and also helps maintain lean muscle mass to improve body composition.

Better blood sugar control: Fasting can not only lower blood sugar, but also increase insulin sensitivity to help your body use insulin more efficiently.

Reduced inflammation: Several studies have shown that fasting can reduce some signs of inflammation, which is thought to play a central role in health and immune function.

Reduces hunger: Intermittent fasting keto can lower levels of leptin, a satiety hormone that signals your brain when it's time to stop eating, and maintaining low leptin levels can help prevent leptin resistance to help control hunger and appetite.

Promotes brain function: Animal studies show that fasting can improve cognitive function and maintain brain health by acting on specific proteins involved in brain aging.

Now you may wonder: how can I do keto and intermittent fasting? With just a few simple steps, it's easy to get started and set yourself up for success.

1. Choose your protocol

There are several different post protocols, making it easy to find a method that works for you. To get started, simply select the protocol that suits your daily life and get started right away. Here are some common methods:

Alternation of posts: This type of food involves fasting every other day. On fasting days, you can opt out of eating altogether or limit your intake to 500 calories per day. On non-hungry days, you should follow a healthy keto diet as usual.

16/8 Post: The 16/8 intermittent ketosis plan consists of fasting for 16 hours a day and limiting food intake to 8 hours a day. This usually means that you don't have to eat anything after dinner and skip breakfast the next morning.

Diet 5: 2: In this plan, you follow a standard keto diet for five days a week and limit your intake to 500-600 calories for the remaining two days.

23/1 Intermittent fasting keto: Using this intermittent fasting method, you should limit your meals to only one hour per day and fast for the remaining 23 hours of the day.

2. Calculate your keto macros

After determining your preferred intermittent fasting protocol, you should start planning your diet for the days you eat. With a standard keto diet, 75 percent of the total calories should come from fats, 20 percent from protein, and 5 percent from carbohydrates. However, when you start, instead you can start with a modified keto diet, which is often considered more flexible and easy to use.

According to this diet, about 40–60 percent of calories should come from healthy keto fats, 20–30 percent from protein foods, and 15–25 percent from carbohydrates.

There are many online calculators that can help determine your daily calorie intake based on factors such as age, gender, and activity level. However, as a rule, men and women need about 2500 calories and 2000 calories per day, respectively, to maintain weight.

3. Make a nutrition plan

Once you have calculated your daily nutrient needs and decided which fasting method is right for you, you can start planning your meals to start keto and intermittent fasting.

Fill your plate with plenty of healthy fats, such as coconut oil, avocados, olive oil, ghee, and grass-fed butter, as well as moderate amounts of protein foods like grass-based meats, poultry, oily fish, and eggs. You can also try non-starchy vegetables, fresh herbs, nuts, seeds and healthy drinks such as water, bone broth and green tea.

4. Get started!

Now that you are properly prepared, it's time to start with a keto periodical. In addition to reducing carbohydrates, increasing fat intake and limiting food intake at a specific time every day, you should also be sure that you need to drink water and plan your workouts according to your fasting schedule.

Although it is good to play sports on days when you are fasting, it is important to listen to your body and avoid excessive effort.

So, how long does it take to switch to ketosis during fasting? On a standard keto diet, it usually takes 2-3 days to achieve ketosis, although in some cases it can take up to seven days.

However, many people believe that intermittent fasting with keto-adaptation can speed up the process and help your body burn glycogen stores faster, causing ketosis.

Keto Post Precautions

Although intermittent fasting and keto can be safe and effective for most, it may not be for everyone.

For example, for people with low blood sugar, long periods without eating can lower blood sugar and cause side effects such as weakness, trembling, and sweating. Therefore, if you have diabetes, you should consult your doctor to determine if you have an intermittent keto on an empty stomach.

Intermittent fasting keto is also not recommended for children, pregnant women, or those with a history of eating disorders. Instead, it's best to focus on a nutrient-rich diet that can help provide the important vitamins and minerals your body needs.

In addition, although many people use periodic fasting keto for bodybuilding, it is best to listen to your body when it comes to fasting and physical activity. Despite the fact that light exercises are usually good, it is recommended to limit the load to 72 hours or more.

Finally, note that fasting causing ketosis can also cause a number of symptoms, often called "keto-flu." Symptoms of fasting with ketosis may include decreased energy levels, increased cravings, digestive problems, muscle pain, and dizziness.

These symptoms can last from a few days to several weeks at the start of a ketogenic diet, but they usually disappear as soon as your body enters ketosis and begins to adapt.

Chapter 5: Intermittent Fasting Diet Plan

Meal plan for seven days

This detox menu of 7 days in total, during the first, second, sixth and seventh days, the body remains, at least, 16 hours without ingesting solids. And the third and fourth days you can fasts completely during the 24 hours.

During fasting, the body responds with detoxification crisis because it is only in the absence of digestion that it can release the accumulated toxins. This, often, is not very pleasant at a symptomatic level, but it is really necessary for later well-being.

In the days in which 16 hours fast during the remaining 8 hours there is food intake, but exclusively with depurative properties, of easy and short digestion so that later the fasting phase is more efficient. These foods are liquid: green smoothies and depurative soups, very nutritious.

The depuration produces positive effects in the short, medium and long term, but at the time it is performed certain symptoms may appear, especially on the second and third days.

If you drink coffee or other exciting, headaches may appear. It is not due to depuration but to abstinence. This symptom can also be triggered in people with a tendency to suffer from migraines. This may be due to the movement of toxins and, in that case, may last beyond the third day.

You can appreciate that the whitish layer that covers the back of the tongue becomes denser. You may notice changes in the taste of the mouth and the density of the saliva. You probably notice that the mouth is drier. They are normal symptoms that the elimination of toxins has already started, and they are reduced with time.

The strong and sweet taste and the smell of the breath indicate that the body is using reserve fats so that the body continues to have energy.

Other changes that can be appreciated are a stronger body odor and darker urine. You will go less to the bathroom. They decrease the stool, and you can suffer constipation the first days. Mild intestinal and stomach discomfort are also normal.

Therefore it is very convenient to follow a diet based on plants the week before detox and then accompany the detox with some colon cleansing treatment (for example, with agar, Zaragoza and other plants with abundant mucilage).

The feeling of lack of energy, which varies greatly from person to person, appears when glucose stores begin to become scarce before the body turns to fat. The available energy is dedicated to elimination and regeneration.

That is why it is important to fast for a few days in which a person can allow a break in physical and mental demands.

7-day detox plan, a menu for each day.

In the first days, you lose weight, which is due to an increase in the elimination of fluids. People with low weight should not do debugging for more than seven days. You can also suffer slight dizziness when getting up from the lying position, as well as cold in the extremities.

Days 1 and 2

When you get up, try to drink a glass of water with the juice of a freshly squeezed lemon.

- Between 11 and 12 h apple juice
- Two apples, preferably granny smith
- ½ lemons with the skin
- Six leaves of cabbage kale
- 1 cup of alfalfa sprouts
- One cucumber
- One piece of ginger to taste
- Two branches of parsley

- ½ celery

- Extract the juice with a slow juice extractor in the order in which the ingredients are listed.

- Around 2:30 p.m. Green smoothie rich in fiber

One bunch of green leaves without the stem (beet leaves, wild leaves, mizuna, and arugula). Mix a maximum of 2 different varieties on the same day. Avoid spinach and chard because of its oxalate content.

- ½ lemon peeled or the juice of 1 lemon

- 1 granny smith apple

- One teaspoon of psyllium husks

- One teaspoon of chlorella

- One piece of turmeric 1 cm

- 150 ml of celery and apple juice or 150 ml of filtered water (you can vary the amount until you get the desired consistency and texture)

- With a high-power mixer, beat all the ingredients until you get the smooth texture of a smoothie.

At 7:00 p.m. Soup with cabbage and celery

- Six cabbage leaves without stems

- One branch of celery with leaves

- ½ avocado

- One teaspoon of chia seeds

- The juice of ½ to 1 lemon

- ½ clove of garlic

- Seven stalks of coriander

- 150 ml of water

- With a high power mixer, mix all the ingredients until you get a fine and creamy texture.

Days 3, 4 and 5

When you get up, always drink a glass of water, but now without the juice so you do not have to sting.

Between 11h and 12h wheatgrass juice

- ½ lemon with the skin
- 1 cup of fresh wheatgrass
- Ten fresh mint leaves
- ¼ celery

Take out the juice with a slow extractor in the same order in which the ingredients are listed. This juice has an unusually low glycemic index, as it has practically no effect on blood sugar levels.

Between 1:30 p.m. And 7 p.m. Juice of cabbage and carrots

- Prepare 3-4 glasses of juice and store it in glass bottles in the fridge. Take one every 2 hours, more or less.
- ½ lemon with the skin
- Six leaves of cabbage kale
- Four carrots
- One beet
- Four radishes
- One piece of ginger to taste
- 1 cup of edible wild leaves

- Two branches of parsley

- ½ celery

- Cut the beet into small dice and pass the ingredients through the slow extractor in the order they appear on this list.

Days 6 and 7

- Between 11 and 12 h wheatgrass juice

- You can see the recipe in the previous section (days 3, 4 and 5).

- Between 1:30 p.m. And 3 p.m. Mint green smoothie

- Six leaves of kale without stem

- ½ peeled lemon or the juice of a lemon

- 1 granny smith apple

- Ten fresh mint leaves

- 150 ml of celery and apple juice or filtered water

Mix the ingredients in the blender until you get a fine and creamy texture. You can vary the amount of liquid ingredients-celery and apple juice, or water-to achieve the desired consistency and texture.

In between 5:30 and 7:00 p.m. Wild leaf detox soup

- One bunch of wild leaves (arugula, canons, dandelion, comfrey, borage, broom, purslane or alfalfa)

- Two celery sticks with leaves

- ½ avocado

- One tablespoon peeled hemp seeds

- The juice of ½ to 1 lemon

- ½ clove of garlic

- Ten leaves of parsley

- 150 ml of water

- Using a high-power mixer beat all the ingredients until the consistency is as fine as possible.

Chapter 6: Intermittent Fasting Recipes

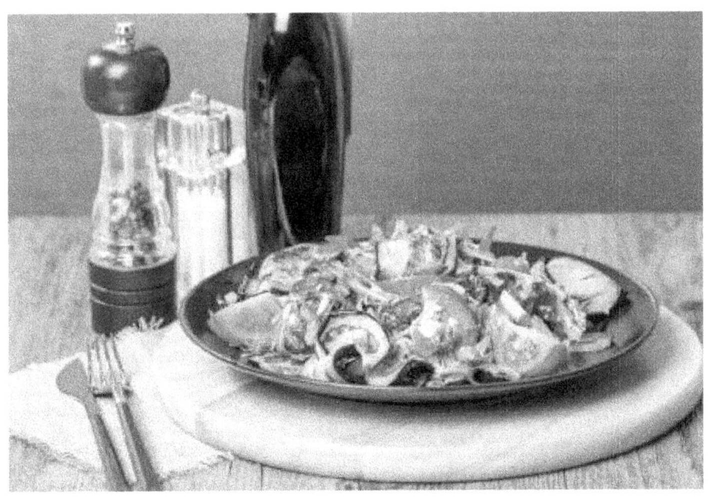

Eggplant salad with spinach grill

Preparation time: 15 minutes

Cooking time: 20 minutes

Ingredients

4 portions

- 1 piece of eggplant sliced and sliced

- 1/8 cup of mint leaves only

- 1/2 bunch of parsley leaves only

- 1 tablespoon of oregano

- 1/4 cup of dehydrated tomato cut in thirds

- 4 cups fresh baby spinach

- 2 cloves garlic, finely chopped, for dressing

- 1 tablespoon of tahini for dressing

- 1/2 tablespoon paprika for dressing

- 1 piece of lemon juice, for dressing

- 1 tablespoon olive oil for dressing

- 1 pinch of salt for dressing

- 1/4 cup of crumbled feta cheese

Preparation

1. Heat a grill over high heat; grill the aubergines until the classic grill marks are formed. Withdraw and reserve

2. In a bowl mix the aubergines with the mint leaves, the parsley, the oregano, the dehydrated tomatoes, and the spinach. Reservation.

3. In a bowl, mix the garlic, tahini, paprika, lemon and olive oil with the balloon whisk and season to your liking.

4. Mix the salad with the dressing and sprinkle to your liking with the feta cheese.

Tip:

The slightly sweet, essentially flowery flavor of marjoram adds a delicate note to this middle eastern-inspired salad, though oregano is also fine. To be assured the eggplant is tender, slice into it before getting it off the grill—when properly prepared, it will be moist all the way through.

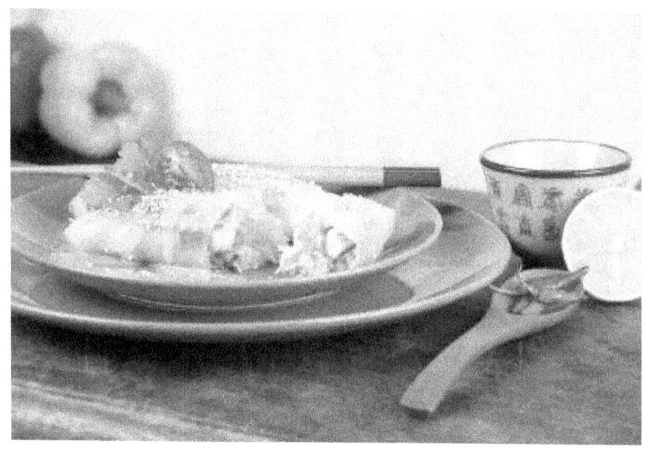

Spring rolls with picosito mango dip

Preparation time: 10 minutes

Cooking time: 20 minutes

Ingredients

10 portions

- 1 cup of water

- 1 tablespoon of rice vinegar

- 5 pieces of rice leaf

- 1/2 cup of alfalfa germ

- 1/2 cup purple cabbage cut into strips

- 1/2 cup fresh coriander leaves

- 2 pieces of carrot cut into canes

- 1 piece of yellow pepper cut into strips

- 1/2 piece of pineapple cut into canes

- 1 piece of handle for the dip

- 1 piece of tree chili

- 1 tablespoon white vinegar

- 1 pinch of salt

- 1 pinch of pepper

- 1 tablespoon garlic powder

Preparation

1. Add to a bowl the water with the rice vinegar; submerge the rice leaves one by one until they have a soft consistency. Reservation.

2. Spread the rice slices in a nonstick plastic add the alfalfa germ, the cabbage, the coriander leaves, the carrot, the yellow pepper, and the pineapple, roll it covering the vegetables well cut in half.

3. Add the mango, the chile de árbol, the white vinegar, the salt, the pepper and the garlic powder to the blender. Blend perfectly well, serve in a bowl and accompany the rolls.

Tip:

Serve the rolls on a plate accompanied by the mango dip.

Cheeseburger lettuce wraps

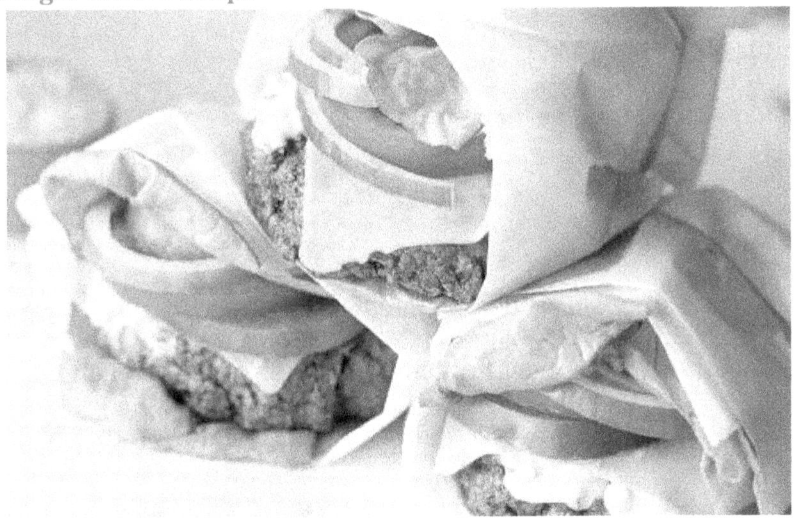

Prep time:23 mins

Ingredients

Select ingredients:

- 2 pounds lean ground beef
- 1/2 teaspoon seasoned salt
- 1 teaspoon fresh ground black pepper
- 1 teaspoon dried oregano
- 6 slices american cheese
- 2 large heads iceberg or romaine lettuce, rinsed then dried
- 2 tomatoes, sliced thin
- Small red onion, sliced thin

Spread:

- 1/4 cup light mayonnaise

- 3 tablespoons ketchup

- 1 tablespoon dill pickle relish

- Dash of salt and pepper

Preparations

1. Preheat a grill or skillet on medium heat.

2. Mix together ground beef, seasoned salt, pepper and oregano.

3. Separate mixture into 6 sections and then roll each into a ball. Flatten balls to form a patty.

4. Place patties on the grill/pan and cook for about 4 minutes on each side.

5. Meanwhile, make the spread. Mix together all of the spread ingredients in a small bowl. Keep in the refrigerator until ready to use.

6. Lay a slice of cheese on top of each burger. Place each burger one end of a large piece of lettuce. Add the spread, one tomato slice, red onion and whatever else you like. Wrap the lettuce up over the top and serve.

Nutrition facts

Servings per recipe

4 servings

Amount per serving

- Calories 300

- Total fat 17g

- Saturated fat 8g

- Trans fat 0.5g

- Cholesterol 95mg

- Sodium 1670mg

- Total carbohydrates 10g

- Fiber 2g

- Sugar 5g

- Protein 27g

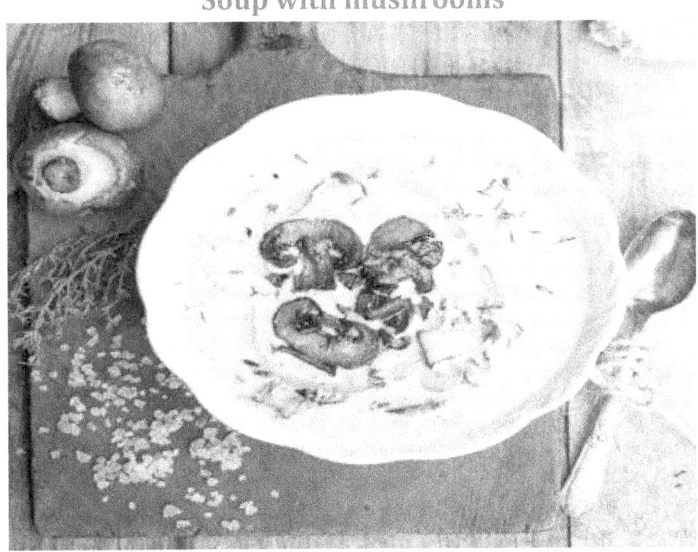
Soup with mushrooms

Ingredients:

For 4 portions | per serving: 185 kcal, 13 g f, 11 g e, 6 g kh

- 2 slices of bacon, cut into 0.5 cm cubes

- 2 tablespoons of shallots or onions, chopped

- 1 teaspoon chopped garlic or the toes of a tuber garlic confit

- 450 g small mushrooms, cleaned and quartered or sliced

- 1 teaspoon dried thyme

- 480 ml chicken bone broth, homemade or bought

- 1 teaspoon fine sea salt

- ½ teaspoon freshly ground

- Black pepper

- 2 big eggs

- 2 tablespoons of lemon juice

For garnish:

- Fresh thyme

- Mct oil or extra virgin olive oil, for drizzling

Preparation:

1. Place the bacon cube in a stock pot and fry over medium heat for about 3 minutes until crispy. Remove the bacon from the pot, but leave the fat in the pot. Put the shallots and garlic in the pan and sauté for about 3 minutes over medium heat until the shallots soften and the garlic begins to smell.

2. Add the mushrooms and dried thyme and cook over medium heat for about 10 minutes until the mushrooms are golden brown. Broth, salt and pepper and bring to a boil.

3. Mix the eggs and lemon juice in a medium sized bowl with the whisk. Continue stirring while slowly adding 120 ml of hot soup (if you add the soup too fast, the egg will clot). Then slowly stir another 120 ml of soup under the egg mixture.

4. Add the hot egg mixture to the stock pot with stirring. Add the fried bacon, then reduce the heat and simmer the keto soup for 10 minutes, stirring frequently. During cooking, the soup will thicken slightly. Remove the pot from the stove and garnish the soup with fresh thyme before serving and drizzle with mct oil.

5. Freshly made keto soup tastes best, but in an airtight container it lasts up to three days in the fridge. To warm up, put the soup in a saucepan and heat over low to medium heat - stirring constantly so that the egg does not clot.

Ice cream with cherry sauce

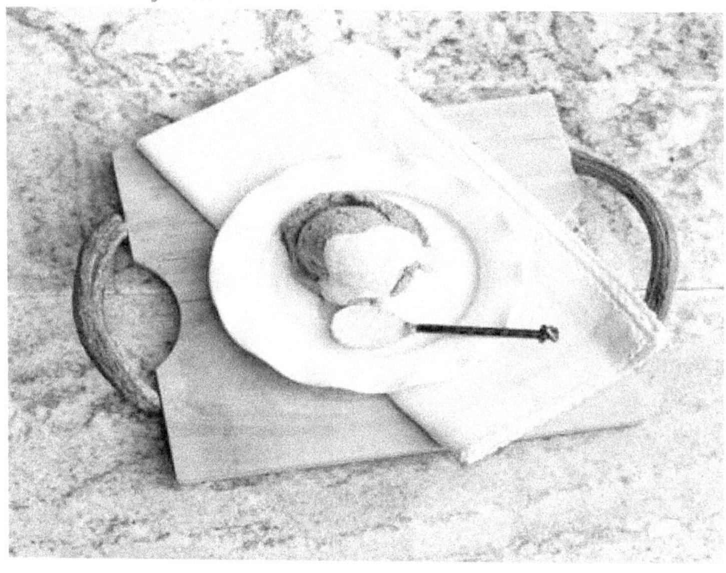

Ingredients:

For 720 ml | per serving (one scoop): 249 kcal, 25.3 g f, 3.5 g e, 2.1 g kh

For the keto ice cream:

- 210 ml of coconut oil or (if tolerated)

- 200 g unsalted butter

- 120 ml unsweetened almond milk or water

- 60 ml of mct oil

- 4 big eggs

- 4 yolks of big eggs

- Freshly scratched pith of a vanilla pod (about 20 cm long) or 1 tsp vanilla extract

- 3 tablespoons finely powdered erythritol

- 1 tsp liquid stevia extract

- 30 g unsweetened cocoa powder

- ¼ teaspoon fine sea salt

For the sauce:

- 1 teabag cherry tea or another fruit tea, if desired b. Raspberry tea

- 120 ml of boiling water

- 3 el erythritol

- ¼ tsp liquid stevia extract

- 60 ml brown butter, room warm, or (in case of intolerance to milk) melted coconut oil

- 1 teaspoon of cherry flavor or, if desired, another fruit flavor, e.g. B. Raspberry flavor

- ⅛ tl guar gum or xanthan gum

Preparation:

1. Add all ingredients for the ice cream to the blender and puree until the mixture is smooth and creamy. Season with erythritol as you like.

2. Add the mass to the icemaker and process into ice cream according to the instructions of the equipment manufacturer.

3. For the sauce, leave the cherry tea in the boiling water for at least 2 minutes. The longer the tea draws, the more intense the fruit taste.

4. Add the cherry tea to the blender and add erythritol, stevia extract, brown butter or coconut oil, and the cherry flavor. Mix everything until a creamy sauce is produced.

5. Mix guar gum or xanthan and leave the sauce for 3 minutes to allow it to thicken.

6. Arrange the chocolate ice cream and add one tablespoon of the still warm cherry sauce.

7. Immediately freeze portions of ice cream in portions in airtight containers and consume within one month.

8. The sauce is not suitable for freezing, but lasts up to four days in the fridge. Heat for 2 to 3 minutes shortly before serving on low heat.

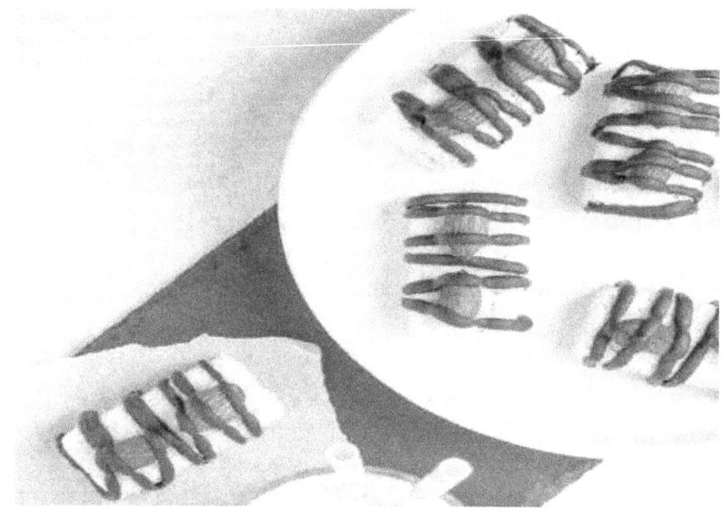

Ingredients:

For 18 keto bars | per serving (one bar): 204 kcal, 18.7 g f, 2.2 g e, 6.6 g kh

- 2 ^{2} / s cups (240 g) unsweetened grated coconut

- 1 serving of sweetened condensed coconut milk, lukewarm

- 1/4 cup (60 ml) of melted coconut oil or ghee (if your diet allows it)

- 1 tbsp plus 1 tsp erythritol

- 1 tsp vanilla extract or powder

- 1/4 teaspoon finely ground gray sea salt

- 36 almonds, roasted

- 1/2 cup (112 g) of stevia sweetened chocolate chips, melted

Preparation:

1. Lay out a baking tray with baking paper or a silicone baking mat. Or, if available, use a silicone muffin mold with 18 rectangular wells (30 ml each).

2. Place the grated coconut, condensed coconut milk, coconut oil, erythritol, vanilla extract and salt in a large bowl and mix thoroughly.

3. When using a baking tray, form 2 tablespoons of dough into a bar with your hands and place on the baking sheet. Repeat the process with the remaining dough. When using a muffin mold, pour 2 tablespoons of dough into each well. In both cases: press the dough well.

4. Put the baking tray or muffin dish in the fridge for at least 30 minutes.

5. Remove the sheet or mold from the refrigerator. If using a muffin mold, carefully lift the keto bars out of the troughs and place on a piece of baking paper or silicone baking mat.

6. Put 2 almonds on each bar and drizzle with melted chocolate.

7. Put the keto bars back in the refrigerator for 15 minutes and then serve.

Note: the bars are in an airtight sealable container in the refrigerator for up to 3 days, in the freezer for up to 1 month. The condensed coconut milk can be prepared up to 3 days in advance and only slightly heated before use in step 2. Almonds can be roasted in large quantities, as they are stable in the freezer for up to 3 months. So they are available quickly.

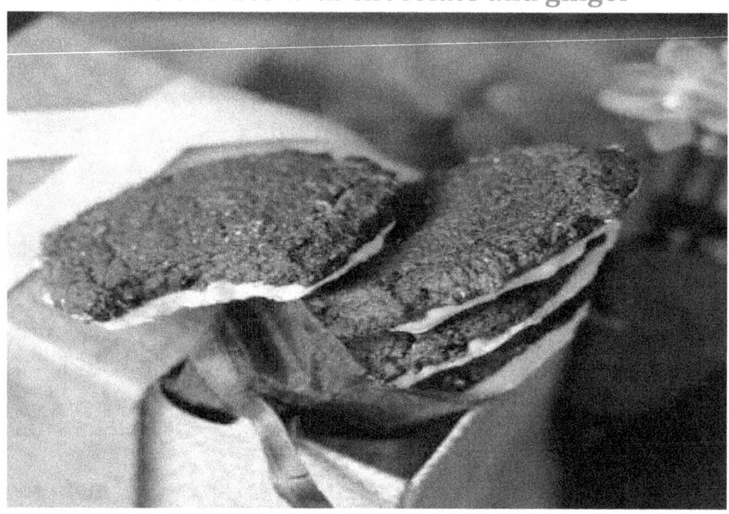

Ingredients:

For 24 keto cookies | per serving (one cookie): 51 kcal, 4.7 g f, 1.1 g e, 1.2 g kh

- 120 g unsalted butter or

- 120 ml coconut oil, room warm

- 220 g finely powdered erythritol or 120 ml yacón syrup

- 1 tsp liquid stevia extract

- 2 big eggs, whisked

- 90 g unsweetened cocoa powder

- 1 tbsp cinnamon

- 2 teaspoons ginger powder

- ¼ teaspoon fine sea salt

- 2 teaspoons of vanilla extract

- ½ teaspoon almond extract

Preparation:

1. Preheat the oven to 175 ° c. Provide two baking trays (do not grease).

2. Place the butter or coconut oil in a mixing bowl and stir frothy, either with a hand mixer or in the food processor. Add erythritol or yacón syrup and stevia extract and stir thoroughly.

3. Stir in the eggs, then add the cocoa powder, cinnamon, ginger powder, salt, vanilla and almond extract and stir the dough again thoroughly.

4. Form the dough into 5 cm balls and place them on the plates at a distance of about 2.5 cm. (the dough diverge when baking.)

5. Bake the cookies for 10 to 12 minutes until they are cooked through. Let cool on the plate.

6. Place the cookies in an airtight container for storage. In the refrigerator they last up to a week, in the freezer up to a month.

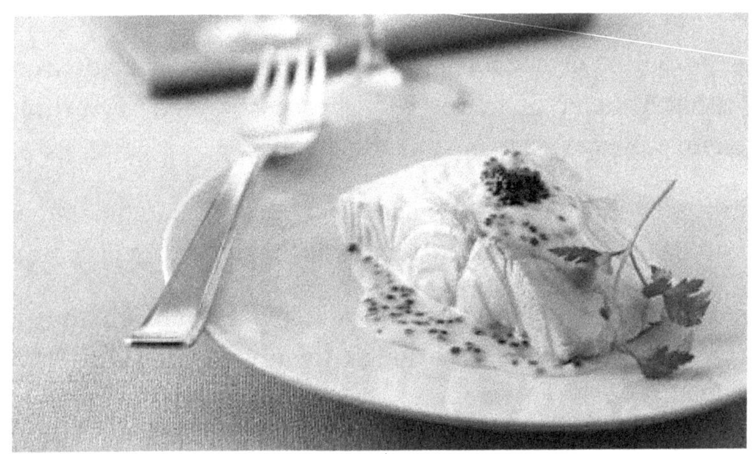

Poached salmon with champagne

Poached salmon with champagne

Preparation time: 10-15 mins

Makes 4 servings

Ingredients

- ➢ 4 salmon fillets (6 ounces each)

- ➢ 1 bottle (740 ml) of brut- type champagne, at room temperature

- ➢ 1 leek or garlic leek (leek), white part only finely cut

- ➢ 1 large shallot, finely chopped

- ➢ 1 lemon cut into wheels

- ➢ Star anise, only one star

- ➢ 6 branches of parsley

> 1 chile serrano cut in half (optional)

> 1 teaspoon salt

> ½ cup of cream (heavy cream)

To decorate

> 1 sprig of parsley

Preparation

1. Pour all ingredients except salmon and cream in a deep pan. Heat over high heat until the mixture boils. Lower to medium heat.

2. Carefully slide the salmon fillets into the champagne mixture. Cover the pan and cook for 4 minutes. Remove the salmon fillets. Do not discard the liquid from the pan.

3. Place ½ cup of the champagne broth in a small saucepan. Heat until it boils and adds the cream slowly. Lower to medium heat and cook, constantly stirring, until thick. Try the sauce and add a pinch of salt, if you like.

4. If the salmon fillets have cooled, reheat the champagne broth and add the salmon fillets. Cook for one or two minutes, or till the salmon, is hot. Remove the fillets from the broth and serve on a plate.

5. Decorate each salmon fillet with a spoonful or two of the cream sauce and a leaf of parsley. Serve with salad or rice.

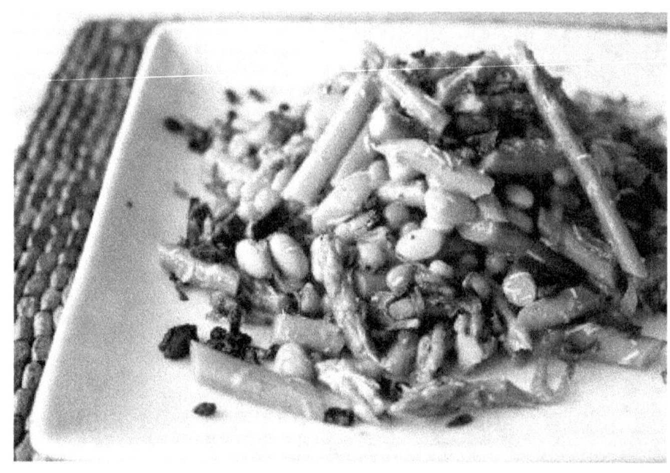

Asparagus and green pea's salad

Green, white or violet, asparagus is consumed in all regions of the world. It is an excellent source of folate, an essential vitamin for pregnant or breastfeeding women. The antioxidants it contains would help our body prevent many diseases.

Ingredients

- ➢ 1/2 of bunch (8 ounces) asparagus
- ➢ 1 1/2 cups of shelled english peas, blanched
- ➢ 1/4 cup of fresh mint leaves (you can tear it, if large)
- ➢ 1/4 cup of chopped toasted almonds, plus more for serving
- ➢ Two tablespoons extra-virgin olive oil
- ➢ Two tablespoons of rice-wine vinegar
- ➢ Kosher salt and freshly ground pepper

Preparation

1. Trim asparagus. Thinly slice on a strong bias. Toss with peas, mint, almonds, oil, and vinegar. Season with salt and then add pepper, and serve, topped with more mint and almonds.

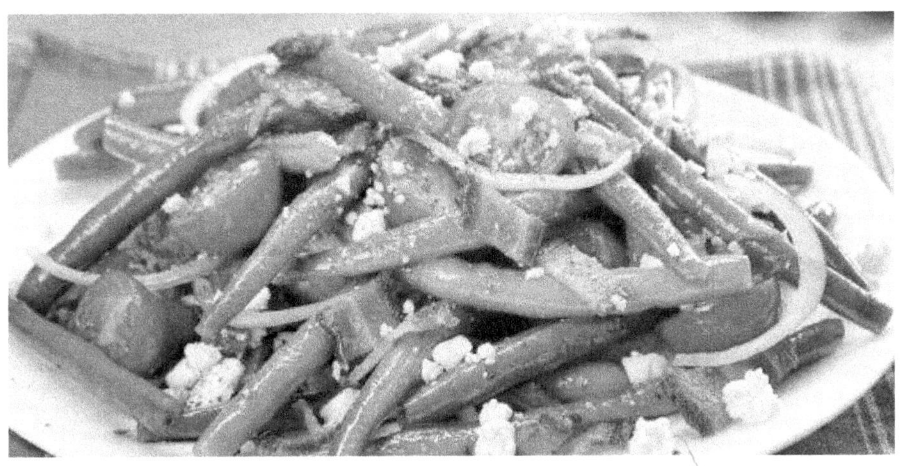

Wilted spinach salad with bacon and balsamic vinaigrette is a fabulous recipe that will make spinach lovers out of those spinach haters. This is an easy-to-make salad with just a few ingredients that makes for a satisfying dish. This salad that doubles as comfort food and impresses your family and friends at the same time.

Ingredients

- Balsamic vinaigrette:
- ¼ cup olive oil
- Three tablespoons balsamic vinegar
- ½ teaspoon finely chopped garlic
- ¾ dijon mustard spoon
- ¾ honey bee teaspoon
- Salt and pepper to taste
- Salad with red grapes, bacon, and walnut:
- 3 cups mixed lettuce (escarole, french, ball, italian)
- ½ cup red grapes, in halves
- Two slices of bacon, golden brown

- ➢ 8-10 praline or natural walnuts
- ➢ Two tablespoons blue cheese, roquefort or blue cheese

Preparation

1. Balsamic vinegar vinaigrette:

2. Mix all ingredients in a jar, cup or dish and mix well until everything is well incorporated.

3. Add season to taste.

4. Salad with red grapes:

5. Cook the bacon until well browned and cut into medium pieces.

6. Mix the lettuce with half of the balsamic vinaigrette.

7. Place on a plate.

8. Add the red grapes in halves, the bacon in pieces, the blue cheese, and the nuts.

9. Serve with the remaining vinaigrette.

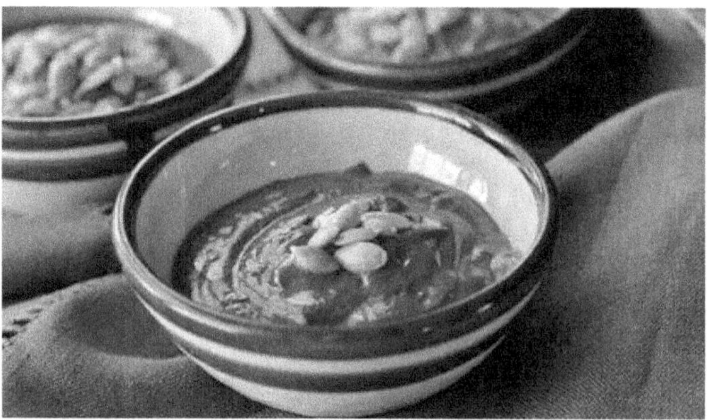

Custard with double chocolate

Preparation time: 10-15 mins

Makes 6 servings

Ingredients

- ➢ 2 cups whole milk
- ➢ 6 tablespoons of sugar
- ➢ 1/4 cup cocoa powder without sugar
- ➢ 2 tablespoons cornstarch
- ➢ 1 1/2 teaspoons cinnamon powder
- ➢ 1/8 teaspoon of salt
- ➢ 2 ounces of bitter chocolate
- ➢ 2 tablespoons toasted pumpkin seeds

Preparation

1. Heat the milk in a microwave in a 1-quart pyrex cup until it almost boils, about 3 to 4 minutes. Meanwhile, beat the sugar, cocoa, cornstarch, cinnamon, and salt in a medium saucepan. At medium heat, add the milk and beat the mixture vigorously. Continue beating until the mixture reaches the consistency of the custard, about two minutes.

2. Remove from heat, add chocolate and beat more.

3. Serve hot or pour in an airtight container or in 6 custard cups covered with plastic to avoid a hard layer of cream. Sprinkle the pumpkin seeds on the custard before serving. It can be kept refrigerated for a maximum of 5 days.

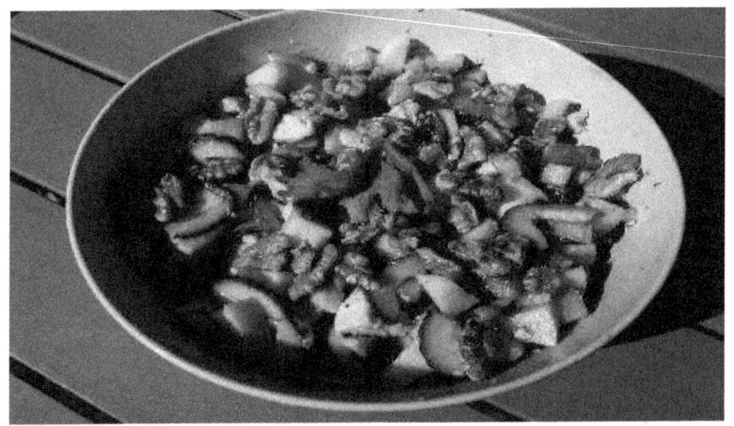

Cucumber salad, cheese and nuts

Preparation time: 15 minutes

Ingredients

- ➢ 100 g of cheese (at least 48% mg)

- ➢ 30 g of nuts

- ➢ 30 g of almonds

- ➢ 1 bag of salad of your choice

- ➢ ½ cup of mushrooms

- ➢ 2 tomatoes

- ➢ ¼ cucumber

- ➢ 4 c. Corn

- ➢ 1 c. Honey coffee

> ➢ 1 c. Mustard

> ➢ 1 c. Tablespoon of coconut oil

Preparation:

1. Cut the mushrooms into strips.

2. Heat the coconut oil inside a pan and fry the mushrooms briefly over high heat.

3. Slice tomatoes, cucumber, and the cheese into small cubes, chop the nuts finely.

4. In a salad bowl, put the tomatoes, cucumber, cheese, nuts, almonds, mushrooms and corn. Stir well.

5. Prepare the vinaigrette by mixing honey, mustard and a little water.

6. Spread the salad on two plates and add the mixture of cheese, nuts, and vegetables.

7. Season with a little vinaigrette and your salad is ready.

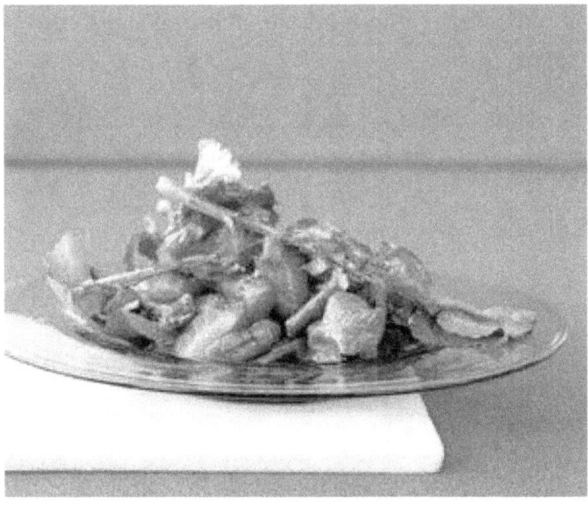

Look for locally grown berries that are brightly colored and plump. They should have the green caps attached and be uniform in size. Avoid soft, shriveled, or moldy fruits. If the strawberries smell sweet, they will most likely taste sweet, too.

Ingredients

- ¼ red onion, thinly sliced
- 4 cups of arugula leaves
- 250 g tapered strawberries
- 90 g goat cheese crumbled
- 1 to 2 cases of balsamic vinegar
- 2 to 3 cases of olive oil
- The salt according to your taste

Preparation

1. Dip the onions in cold, lightly salted water to remove the bitter side.
2. Mix the balsamic vinegar, olive oil and salt in a tight container and shake to the rhythm of the salsa.
3. Drain the onions and mix with the arugula leaves and the vinaigrette.
4. Top with crumbled cheese, sliced strawberries, and spicy pecans.
5. Mix at the table and serve immediately.

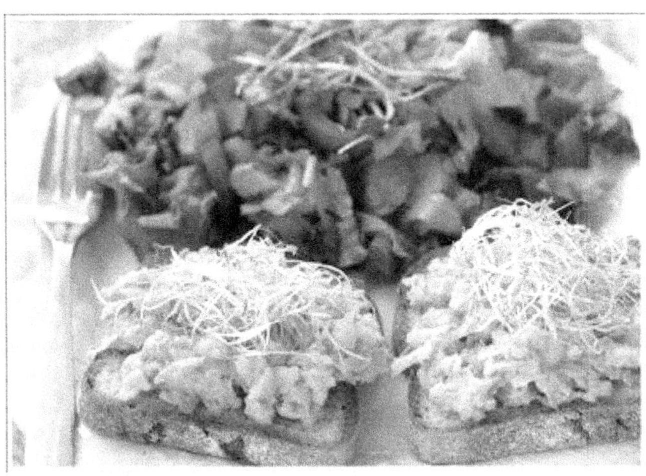

This is a really great tuna salad recipe. The secret ingredients are the curry and parmesan cheese. Odd combinations but this makes a terrific tuna sandwich. It is used as an appetizer with gourmet crackers and people always wanted this recipe.

Ingredients

- 400 g natural tuna one beautiful romaine 100 g raisins two medium pippin apples one lemon juice one teaspoon curry 1 cup mayonnaise

Preparation of the tuna salad with curry:

1. Open the can of tuna. Drain and divide into large pieces.

2. Wash and dry the salad leaves thoroughly. Peel apples before cutting into thin slices sprinkle the lemon juice to prevent them from turning black.

3. Dressing the tuna salad with curry:

4. In a salad bowl, arrange the salad leaves, the pieces of tuna, the raisins and the slices of apple to mix everything.

5. Add the curry to the mayonnaise and stir well.

6. Mix the mayonnaise with the salad just before serving.

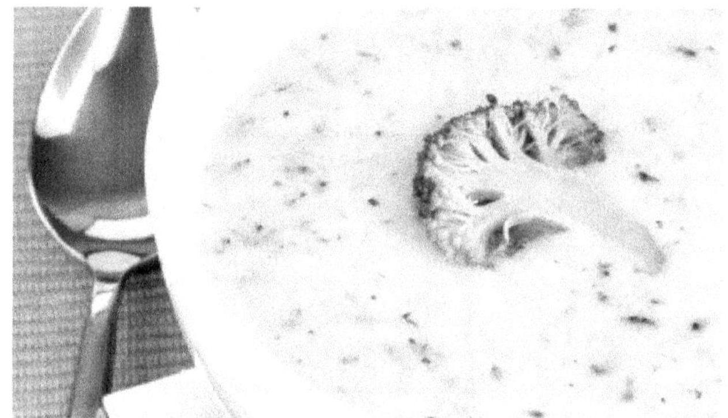

Broccoli, zucchini & onions soup: super healthy recipe

Preparation time: 10-15 mins

Ingredients

- ➤ 150 g broccoli
- ➤ ½ courgette
- ➤ ½ red onion
- ➤ 1 c. Tablespoon of coconut oil
- ➤ 400 ml of water
- ➤ 1 bouillon-cube with herbs

Preparation:

1. Cut the red onion and zucchini into small pieces.

2. Then cut the broccoli florets.

3. Heat the coconut oil inside a pan and fry the red onion for about 3 minutes. Then cook the zucchini for 5 minutes.

4. Add the broccoli florets, water, and bouillon cube. Simmer on low heat for 4 minutes.

5. Reduce everything to the blender until you get a creamy soup.

6. This broccoli, zucchini and onion soup can be served immediately or reheated later as you wish. Enjoy your meal!

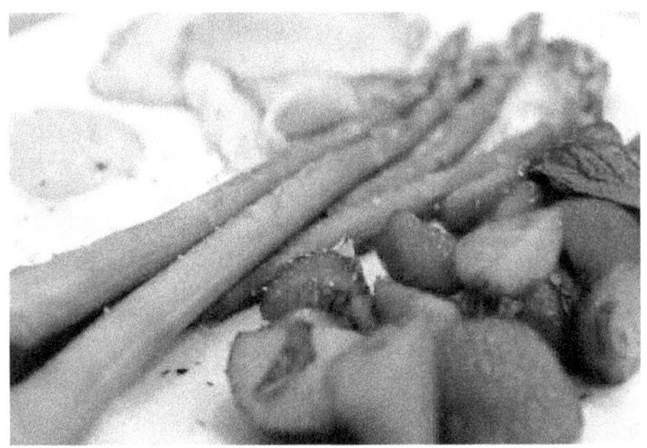

Mint strawberries with green asparagus

Ingredients

For 2-3 persons

- ➤ 1000 g asparagus (green)

- ➤ 500 g strawberries

- ➤ 2-3 fried eggs

- ➤ 250 g of ham (e.g., farmer's ham, cooked ham, etc.)

- ➤ Some branches of fresh mint

➢ Salt pepper

Preparation

1. Wash the asparagus and then slice off the ends (woody taste).

Tip for women between 40 - 65:

There is a special program for interval fasting during menopause! The interval fast is combined with nutritional plans, so that the female body, despite the "menopause hormone conversion" goes back into the fat burning mode.

2. Wash the strawberries, cut the stalk and halve or quarter as desired. Slice the mint and then mix it with the strawberries.

3. Use a large pot of salted water to the boil, add the asparagus, bring to a boil and cook over medium heat for 5-7 minutes.

4. Heat a pan with butter and fry the fried eggs over medium heat and lid.

5. Hams are enough.

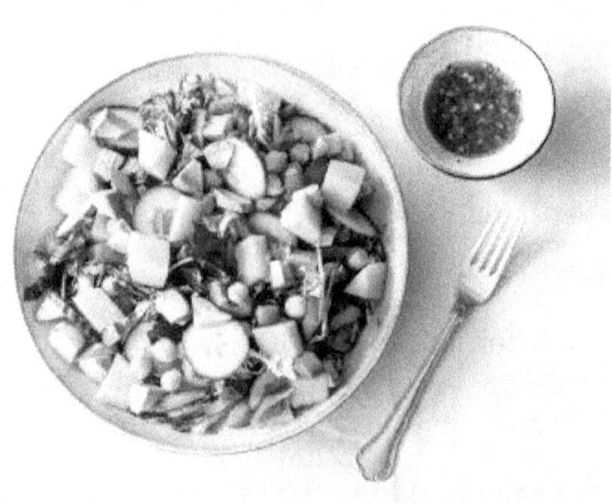

This quick-curry recipe jazzes up cooked beets within minutes. Mixing the beet's earthy sweetness with citrus and a hint of curry spice is a delicious combination. Plus - beets, curry, and walnuts are quite nutritious offering incredible health benefits.

Curry powder and leaves may help protect against heart disease, reduce alzheimer's disease symptoms, ease inflammation, boost the immune system, and remove toxins from the body. These are some of the many reasons (besides the fabulous taste) to pump up the "heat".

High in plant-based omega-3 fats, walnuts are delicious nutrient-dense nuts that may help improve cardiovascular function, balance weight control, and improve brain function. Toasted walnuts also provide a great balance to beets and lemon juice.

This curried beet and toasted walnut salad pairs well with rice (brown, white, or jasmine whichever you prefer).

Ingredients:

- Qs beetroot
- Qs of apples
- Qs chicken breast
- Classic curry vinaigrette
- Nuts and nuts
- Salt and freshly ground pepper

Preparation:

1. Salt the chicken breasts and cook in a drizzle of oil. Book them 5 minutes.
2. Peel the beets, and grate them with a robot or julienne with a mandolin.

3. Cut the apples into fine julienne with a mandolin or knife, or dice to make it easier. You can peel them first reserve the julienne or the dice in the refrigerator.

4. Prepare classic vinaigrette by adding curry powder, and season the beets.

5. Arrange the beets on the plate add the diced apples or julienne and crushed hazelnuts.

6. Slice or dice the chicken breasts and add them to the beets.

7. It's ready to eat.

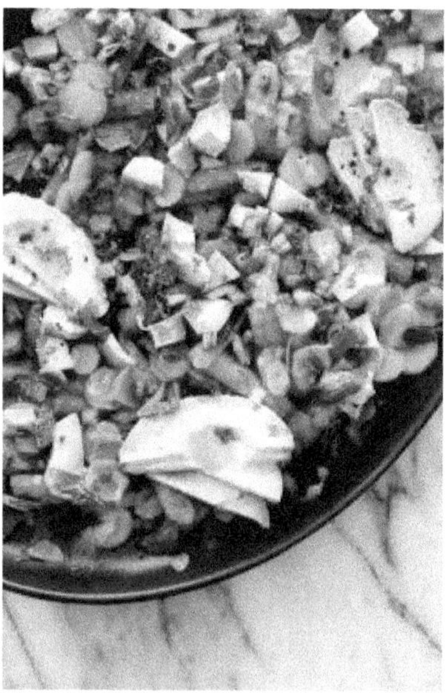

Roasted carrots and cashew salad on lemon vinaigrette

The crunchy texture of sliced red cabbage, paired with the sweet flavor of roasted carrots and lots of chopped parsley, makes a pretty great salad. But when these ingredients are tossed with a flavorful creamy dressing, this simple salad is taken to another level.

The dressing gets its creamy consistency from raw cashew butter the neutral flavor is perfect in dressings as it helps carry flavor without overpowering it. (the cashew butter can be easily replaced with tahini for the same consistency and a pronounced sesame flavor.) The bright, tangy flavor of the dressing comes from good-quality, unpasteurized apple cider vinegar it's worth seeking out to use in any salad dressing, and it's especially helpful to have around when you're out of lemons.

Ingredients / for 2 people

> Four beautiful carrots

> One wrist of cashew nuts

> One wrist of parsley or coriander

> One tablespoon soup grape dry

> For seasoning:

> One lemon

> One tablespoon of tahini

> Two tablespoons of olive oil

> One tablespoon of hazelnut oil

Preparation

1. Peel the carrots and grate them. Put them on a serving plate. Mince the parsley and add to the carrots. Add the raisins on top.

2. Heat 1 tablespoon of vegetable oil in a skillet over high heat and sauté the cashews. Stir frequently, so they do not burn. When they turn a beautiful golden color, place them on paper towels and salt them. Let them cool before adding them to the carrots.

3. Prepare the seasoning: squeeze the lemon and place the juice in a bowl. Add the tablespoon tahini and mix well with a fork to fully dilute the sesame puree. Add two tablespoons of olive oil with a tablespoon of hazelnut oil. Mix the sauce well to incorporate the oils.

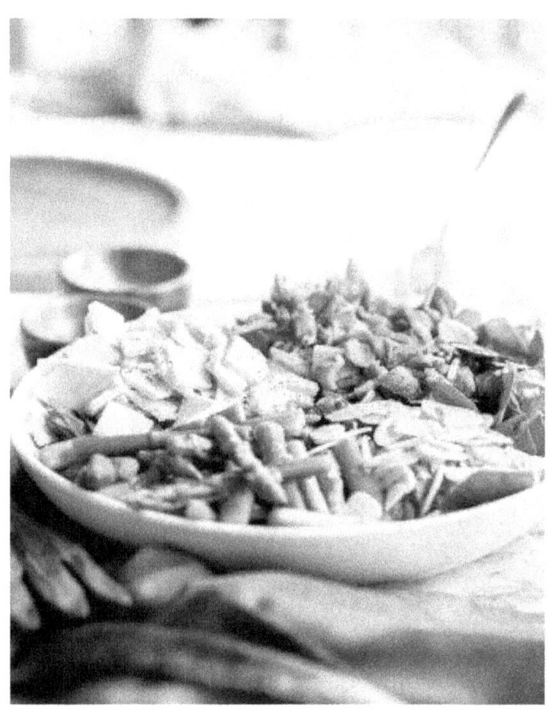

Baby spinach, chicken and carrot salad

Baby spinach, chicken and carrot salad with red wine is at the very top of most super food lists because the many vitamins and minerals it contains, which give it the ability to help prevent disease and provide a multitude of other nutritional benefits. This recipe will explore the health benefits of spinach leaves and why it's good to put this leafy green on your grocery list.

Leafy green vegetables, especially spinach, contain more nutrients than virtually any other vegetable. A mere cup of cooked spinach contains only 41 calories and has exceptionally high levels of vitamins k and a. The vegetable also contains high percentages of the daily values of other vitamins and minerals.

Ingredients

- ➤ Carrots: 2
- ➤ Red onions: 3

- ➢ Spinach sprouts: 80 g

- ➢ Olive oil: 3 tbsp. Soup

- ➢ Lemon juice: 0.5 tbsp. Coffee

- ➢ Juice of 1/2 orange

- ➢ Agave syrup: 1 tbsp. Coffee

Preparation

1. Peel the carrots and onions. Cut the carrots into slices using a thrifty knife and sliced onions.

2. Wash the spinach sprouts, and then drain them. Mix in a medium bowl with the carrots and onions.

3. Mix the agave syrup with the olive oil and the orange and lemon juice. Pour over the salad and mix before serving. Enjoy it immediately.

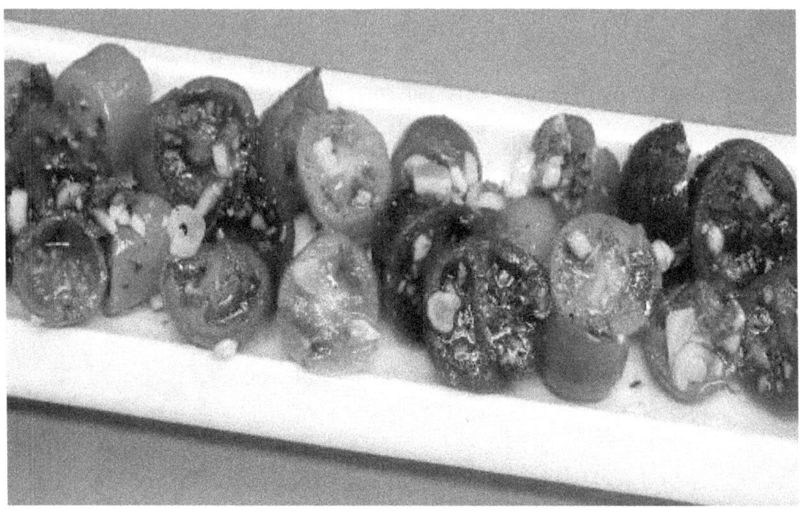

Plum tomatoes and peppers salad

A tomato is a nutrient-dense super food that offers benefit to a range of bodily systems. Its nutritional content supports healthful skin, weight loss, and heart health.

Ingredients

- ➢ Green peppers: 2
- ➢ Red peppers: 2
- ➢ Yellow peppers: 2
- ➢ Cherry tomatoes: 400 g
- ➢ Yellow lemon: 1
- ➢ Olive oil: 5 cl
- ➢ Bouquet of parsley dish: 1
- ➢ Red onion: 1
- ➢ Salt
- ➢ Pepper

Preparation

Take off the first skin of your bunion and chisel it.

Wash your peppers. Cut them in 2, eliminate the peduncles, the seeds as well as the white dimensions. Cut the flesh into small cubes.

Wash and cut your cherry tomatoes in 2 or quarters according to their sizes.

In a salad bowl, mix the tomatoes with the peppers, the onion, the juice of your lemon, the olive oil, salt, and pepper.

Chop the parsley.

Serve your salad by garnish with parsley.

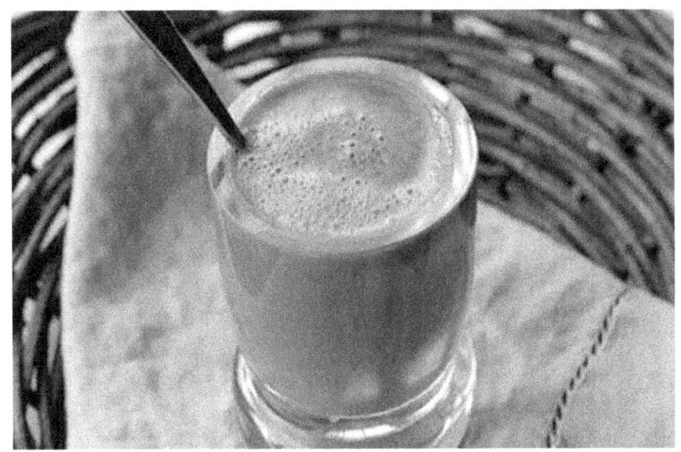

Hot chocolate with coconut

Makes 2 servings

Do not confuse the coconut drink with milk or canned coconut cream. The coconut drink is almost always found in the non-dairy milk section.

Ingredients

- 2 cups of coconut drink (like coconut dream)
- 2 ounces of bitter chocolate
- 1 pinch of salt
- 1 teaspoon vanilla extract

Preparation

Mix the coconut drink, chocolate, and salt and simmer the mixture in a medium saucepan, whisking until the chocolate melts. Remove from heat, add vanilla and serve.

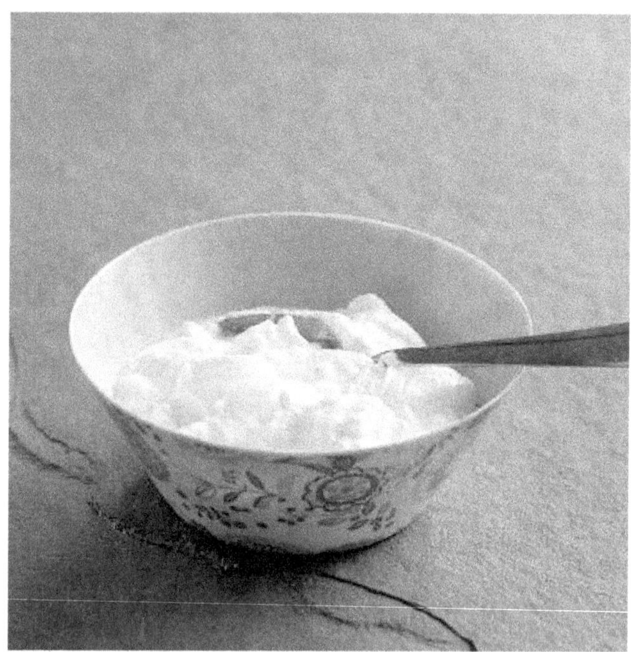

Preparation time: 30 min

Ingredients

- 1 l of pasteurized whole milk

- 100 ml of bought thick milk

Preparation

Put the milk in a bowl or a wide jug. Stir in the used milk with the whisk and let the milk stand at room temperature for approx. 20 hours and let it thicken. Then it can be spooned or drunk or enriched with fruit without any further ingredients.

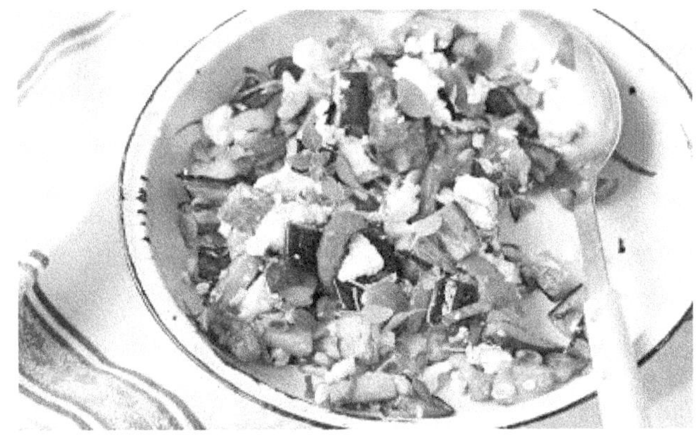

Eggplants contain powerful antioxidant phenols, which are important for neutralizing damaging free radicals in your body. Red bell peppers are the richest dietary source of vitamin c. Just one small bell pepper may provide up to 123% of the recommended daily allowance (rda).

Pine nuts are comprised of numerous health promoting phytochemicals, vitamins, antioxidants, and minerals that have anti-aging effects & may benefit vision and heart health. Research also shows pine nuts can help in suppressing your appetite! Enjoy this healthy and delicious recipe.

Ingredients for the salad are

- One tablespoon of coriander seeds
- One teaspoon of cumin seeds
- Two eggplants of (aubergines), peeled and cut into large chunks
- Two tablespoons of olive oil, plus extra for frying
- Two garlic of cloves
- Gluten-free flour, for dusting
- ⅔ cup (3½ oz/100 g) pine nuts
- One bunch parsley leaves coarsely well chopped

- A handful of baby spinach leaves, chopped

- A handful of pomegranate seeds

- Salt and pepper

- For the dressing

- Four tablespoons pomegranate juice

- One teaspoon balsamic vinegar

- Juice ½ lemon

- Four tablespoons of olive oil

- Salt and pepper

Preparation

Preheat the oven to about 200 º c gases.

Put the coriander and cumin seeds in a deep mortar and then crush them with a pestle. Toast them into a dry skillet or frying pan for a few minutes, or until fragrant.

Put the eggplants (aubergines) in a large bowl and toss with olive oil, crushed garlic, salt, and with pepper then sprinkle on the toasted coriander and cumin seeds.

Drizzle one tablespoon of oil onto a baking sheet. Then dip the eggplants lightly in the flour. Place them all onto the baking sheet and then roast for 30 minutes, or until chargrilled and slightly crisp. Let cool.

While the eggplants are there roasting, mix all the dressing ingredients and set aside.

Put the roasted eggplants into a medium bowl, pour 1–2 tablespoons of the dressing, and toss well. Let stand for about 10 minutes so that the dressing can be absorbed.

Heat 2 teaspoons of olive oil into a skillet and lightly toast the pine nuts until it appears golden.

Add the chopped parsley, spinach, and then pomegranate seeds to the eggplants and toss them all together well. Sprinkle the toasted pine nuts and serve with the remaining dressing.

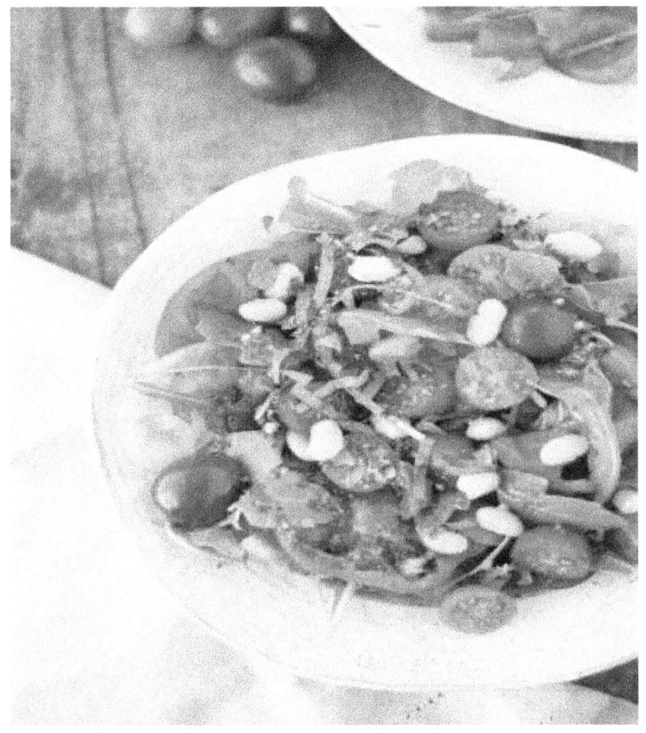

Ripe tomatoes and basil salad

In case you were wondering, a tomato is a technically a fruit, because it's seed-bearing and develops from the ovary of a flowering plant. (botanically speaking, vegetables consist of other plant parts, like roots, leaves, and stems.) But when it comes to nutrition, tomatoes along with seedy cucumbers and zucchini are categorized as vegetables. That's due in part to their lower carb and sugar contents: a medium tomato provides just 22 calories, and about 5 grams of total carb, with 3 as sugar and 1.5 as fiber. But this low-calorie, low-carb package is chock-full of nutrients, and has been linked to a variety of health benefits.

Ingredients

Serves: 2

- Four vines ripened tomatoes
- Good pinch sea salt
- Handful basil leaves rolled and thinly sliced
- One tablespoon good aged balsamic vinegar
- One tablespoon extra-virgin olive oil

Preparation

Prep: 5min

Ready in 5min

Grab an attractive serving plate; flat glass or black works nicely. Slice the tomatoes thinly and scatter onto a plate. Sprinkle with salt, then spread all over the basil leaves. Drizzle over the vinegar and oil. Cover with cling film and then leave at room temperature until ready to serve.

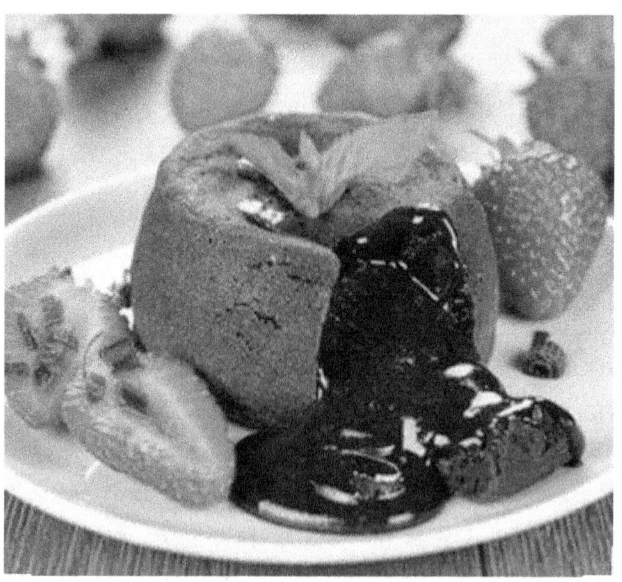

Makes 4 servings

Ingredients

- ➢ 6 ounces semiamargo chocolate (70% cocoa)

- ➢ 8 ounces of cold, thick cream (keep it in a container with ice)

- ➢ ½ teaspoon of instant espresso coffee

- ➢ Oz butter, soft or at room temperature

- ➢ Tablespoons of orange liqueur (or whatever you like)

- ➢ ½ cup of granulated sugar

- ➢ 1 tablespoon of powdered sugar

    - ➢ 3 separate eggs, yolks and whites

    - ➢ Pinch of salt

To decorate

- ➢ 1 teaspoon chocolate scrape

- ➢ 4 strawberries cut in a fan shape

Preparation

1. Melt chocolate with butter and espresso coffee in a bain-marie over medium-low heat, mixing continuously. Once it melts, put it aside.

2. Place the yolks and a quarter of a cup of sugar in a glass vessel in a bain-marie; mix with the grinder while the water is heated over low, medium heat. Mix for a few minutes or until the yolks are warm. Continue moving until the sugar dissolves.

3. Remove from the heat and then continue stirring with the hand blender until it has a creamy consistency (almost like mayonnaise). Put aside.

4. Place the three egg whites and the remaining sugar cube in a bain-marie glass bowl and mix with the grinder, while the water is heated to medium-low heat. Mix until the whites are warm and the sugar dissolves.

5. Remove from heat, add a pinch of salt and stir with a hand blender until you get a consistency of hard meringue.

6. Place the creamy yolks on the side of the container that contains the meringue and incorporates them into the mixture in an enveloping form.

7. Add the chocolate on one side of the container and incorporate it into the mix in an enveloping form.

8. Beat the cream, powdered sugar, and orange liqueur to the point of hard meringue and integrate it, in an enveloping form, into the mixture that the chocolate already contains.

9. Place mousse in glasses and garnish with strawberries and chocolate scrape. To enjoy!

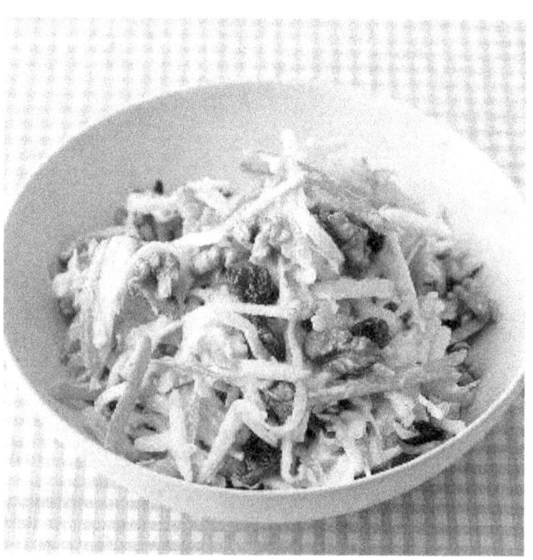

Curry celery salad with honey

Preparation time: 30 min

For 2 servings

Ingredients

> ➢ 1 small celeriac (about 300 g)
>
> ➢ 2 carrots (about 200 g)
>
> ➢ 2 short apples (about 320 g)
>
> ➢ 70 g walnut kernels
>
> ➢ 500 g of yogurt
>
> ➢ 1 tbsp rapeseed oil
>
> ➢ 2 teaspoons curry powder
>
> ➢ 2-3 tablespoons of orange juice
>
> ➢ 1 tsp honey
>
> ➢ 50 g raisins
>
> ➢ Salt
>
> ➢ Pepper

Preparation

1. Wash celery and carrots and peel. Wash, quarter and core the apples. Crush everything in the lightning chopper or grate it roughly with the grater. Chop walnuts roughly as desired.

2. Mix the yogurt with oil, curry powder, orange juice, and honey and mix with raisins and the remaining ingredients: salting and peppering.

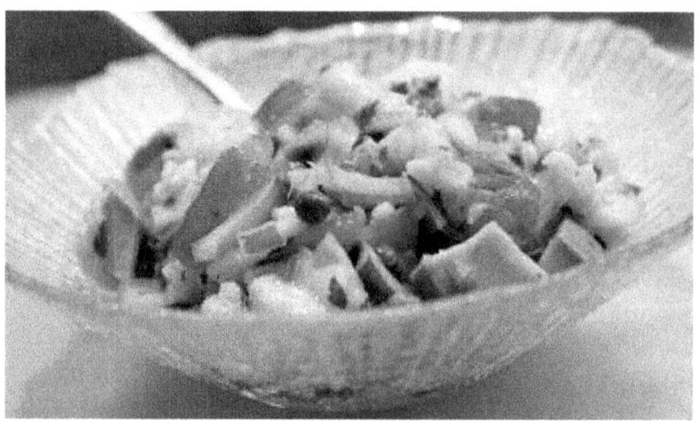

Tilapia ceviche

Makes 6 servings

Ingredients

- ➢ 2 pounds of top quality tilapia, cut in cubes

- ➢ 14 limes (green lemons), cut in halves, plus 1 additional cut into slices, to garnish

- ➢ ½ cup chopped tomato, without seeds

- ➢ ½ cup chopped cucumber, seeded

- ➢ 1/3 cup finely chopped onion

- ➢ ¼ cup fresh chopped cilantro

- ➢ Salt and freshly ground black pepper

- ➢ ½ cup of tomato juice and clams (optional)

- ➢ 1 tablespoon hot sauce bottle (optional)

- ➢ Grilled toast on the grill

- ➢ Mayonnaise to spread

➤ 1 avocado (avocado), peeled, seedless and cut into thin slices

Preparation

1. Place the tilapia inside a medium bowl size. Squeeze the juice out from the lime halves over fish and then mix carefully to combine. Cool in the refrigerator until the fish turns completely white, about 15 minutes.

2. Squeeze the fish with your hands thoroughly to drain the lime juice. Discard the lime juice. Add tomato, cucumber, onion, and cilantro, and mix.

3. Season with salt and pepper to taste.

4. If you wish, add the tomato and clam juice and the hot sauce.

5. Spread mayonnaise generously on toast. Add the ceviche on toast. Place the avocado slices over the ceviche and serve immediately with the slices of lime.

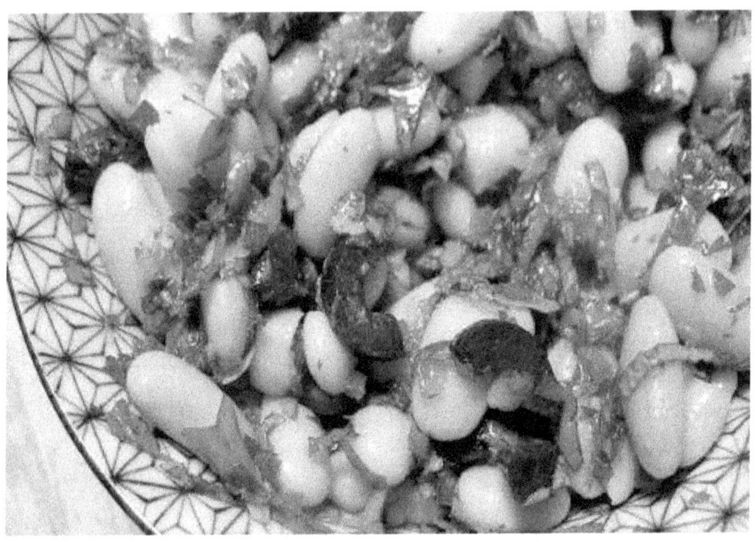

Beans salad

Ingredients

- ➢ 2 pounds of ground beef from animals fed pasture (17% fat)
- ➢ 2 cups chopped onion
- ➢ 2 tablespoons chopped garlic cloves
- ➢ 1 medium jalapeño pepper, chopped, without seeds or veins
- ➢ 1½ tablespoons chili powder
- ➢ 2 teaspoons ground cumin
- ➢ 7 whole tomatoes, chopped
- ➢ 2 cups of tomato sauce
- ➢ 1 1/2 cup red beans or drained and washed beans
- ➢ 1/4 cup of plain yogurt or low-fat yogurt
- ➢ 1/4 cup grated cheddar cheese from pasture-fed animals, or low-fat cheddar cheese from pasture-fed animals

Preparation

Heat a large 5-liter pot. Add the minced beef. Cook, stir and separate the meat, until golden brown. Drain the excess fat, and leave a small amount to cook the onions in it.

Add the onion and cook for about 5 minutes. Add the garlic and jalapeño; cook until tender. Add the chili powder and cumin. Continue cooking until they release odor, approximately 1 minute.

Add the ground tomatoes and the tomato sauce. Cook over low heat for about 30 minutes.

Add the beans and continue cooking, uncovered, until the meat and beans are very soft and the chili is thick, about 30 minutes more. Serve in small bowls. Garnish each bowl with 1 tablespoon of yogurt and cheddar cheese.

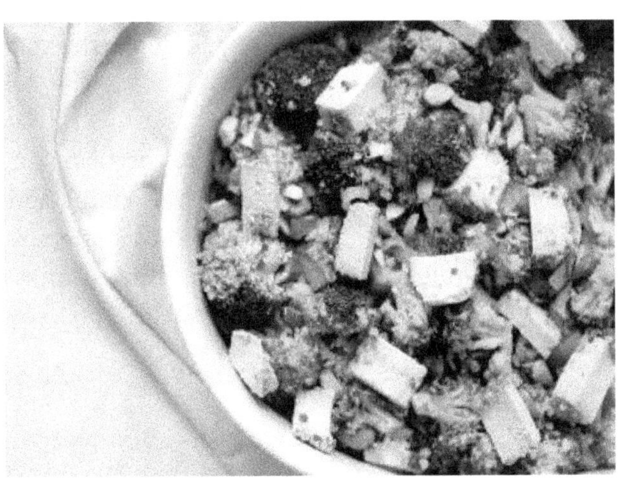

Tofu and broccoli salad

Sauce

- ½ cup (125 ml) water

- 125 ml (½ cup) of hoisin sauce

- ➢ 1 cinnamon stick

- ➢ 4 star anis

- ➢ Jumped up

- ➢ 454 g (1 lb.) Firm tofu, diced

- ➢ ¼ cup (60 ml) canola oil

- ➢ 1 broccoli, cut into small bunches

- ➢ 1 onion, finely chopped

- ➢ 2 cloves of garlic, chopped

- ➢ 1/3 cup (75 ml) unsalted peanuts, toasted and crushed

Preparation

1. Sauce

2. In a saucepan, bring to the boil all the ingredients. Simmer for about 3 minutes or until the sauce is slightly syrupy. Remove the spices. Book.

3. Jumped up

4. In a large pan, brown the tofu in the oil. Add broccoli and cook for about 5 minutes on medium heat or until broccoli is al dente. Add the onion and garlic and sauté for 2 minutes. Add the sauce and mix well. Continue cooking for about 2 minutes. Serve on rice vermicelli. Garnish with peanuts.

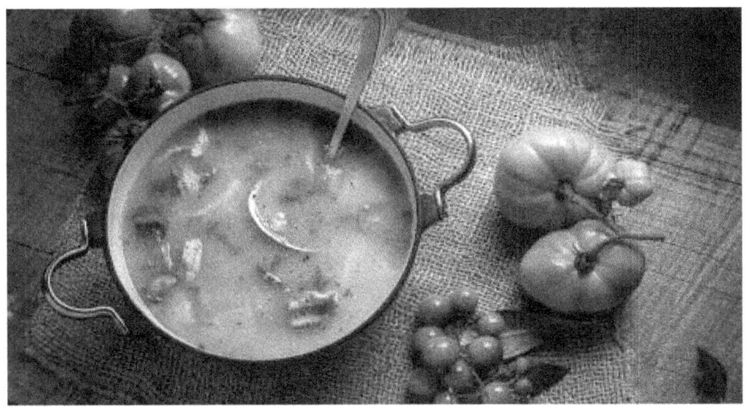

Grouper in green sauce

A soft and delicious low-calorie fish easy to prepare and serve in green tomatillo sauce

Yield: 2 servings

Ingredients

- ➢ 2 grouper fillets
- ➢ Salt and pepper
- ➢ 1 tablespoon of olive oil

For the sauce:

- ➢ 2 tomatillos, without the peel
- ➢ ¼ cup of pumpkin seeds
- ➢ ½ cup of green paprika, without seeds or veins
- ➢ ½ cup of coriander leaves only
- ➢ ½ of a jalapeño, without seeds or veins
- ➢ ½ cup of parsley leaves only

- ➢ ½ teaspoon fresh thyme

- ➢ 3 garlic cloves

- ➢ ¼ cup of fish stock

- ➢ 1 pinch of salt

Preparation:

1. In a medium saucepan with water at the time, add the tomatillos and boil 1 minute. Stir and place in the blender.

2. In a medium skillet, add the seeds and toast on low, medium heat for 1 to 2 minutes or until golden brown. Remove and place in the blender.

3. Pour the rest of the ingredients. Blend well.

4. Pour out the sauce into the pan and then cook over medium heat for 1 minute.

5. Dry the fish fillets with the paper towel and salt and pepper to taste.

6. In another wide pan, add the olive oil and let it heat over medium-high heat.

7. Place the steaks and let them brown, 3 to 4 minutes on each side. Serve with the sauce.

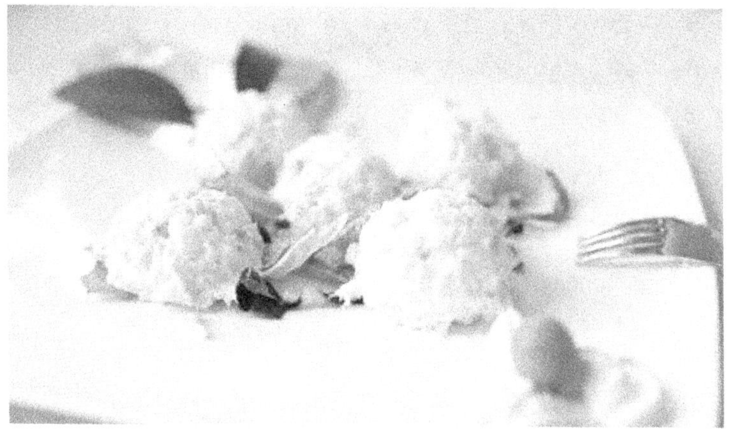

Creamy cod, italian style

Makes 4 servings

Ingredients

> 1 pound, 5 ounces of cod, soaked in water the night before and drained

> ⅔ cup of olive oil

> 1 small onion finely chopped

> ½ cup of milk

> Salt and pepper to taste

Preparation

1. Put the cod inside a medium saucepan and cover with water. Cook over average-high heat until it reaches the boiling point, and then cook over low heat for about 25 more minutes. Turn off the heat, drain the cod and let it cool. Once it's cold, crumble it and remove the thorns, if you have it.

2. Inside a large skillet, heat a little olive oil and cook the onion over medium heat until translucent. Add the cod and the rest of the olive oil.

3. While cooking the cod heat the milk in a small pot over low heat, let it boil. Turn off the heat and then slowly add it to the pan with the cod, beating the mixture vigorously, but carefully, to incorporate all the ingredients well.

4. Cook the cod over low heat for one hour until the mixture is creamy and thick — season with salt and pepper to taste.

5. Serve with rice, polenta or vegetables.

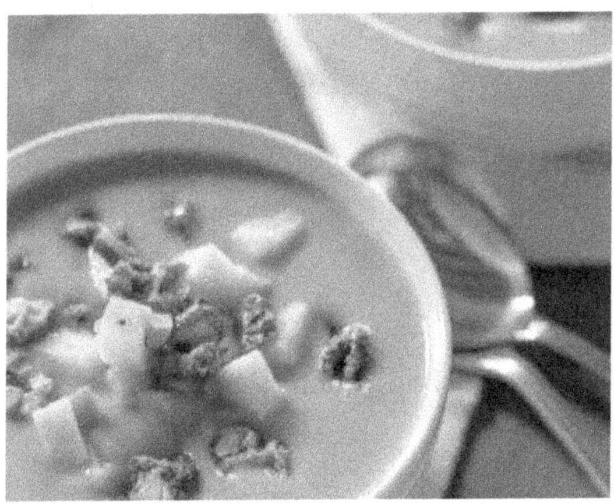

Pumpkin and apple soup

Pumpkin is low in calories, rich in belly-filling fiber and is an excellent source of vitamin a. Using pure canned pumpkin seriously cuts down on prep time, but if you are feeling extra ambitious, roasting or steaming then mashing your own pumpkin would be delicious.

Ingredients

> 450 grams (1 lb.) Pumpkin

> 1 granny smith apple cored, and quartered

> One medium onion cut

> Two cloves garlic

> One tablespoon of olive oil

- ➢ Salt

- ➢ ¼ teaspoon of cayenne more to taste

- ➢ 300 ml (1¼ cup) of vegetable stock

- ➢ Freshly ground black pepper to add taste

Garnish:

- ➢ Pomegranate arils

- ➢ Some pumpkin seeds

- ➢ Fresh parsley finely chopped

Preparation

Preheat the oven about 200 degrees c (or 392 degrees f). Line a large baking sheet with a parchment paper.

Cut the pumpkin half lengthways and scoop out seeds.

Slice each pumpkin half in half to make quarters and place, cut-side up, on a baking tray, along with the onions.

Drizzle with olive oil and then sprinkle some salt.

Bake for about 20 minutes, then add the garlic and apple, flip the pumpkin cut side down and then roast for another for 20 minutes, or until the flesh is soft.

Use a spoon to scoop out the flesh of the pumpkin and transfer to a high-speed blender with the apple, onion, garlic (remove the skins), cayenne, and vegetable stock.

Blend on high for almost 2 minutes, or until silky smooth.

If too thick, add vegetable stock to thin it out and blend over. Taste and adjust the seasonings.

Serve, ladle soup into a bowl, and with pomegranate arils, pumpkin seeds, fresh parsley and freshly ground black pepper.

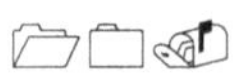 Then serve.

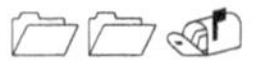 Refrigerate leftovers in an airtight container for 4 days,

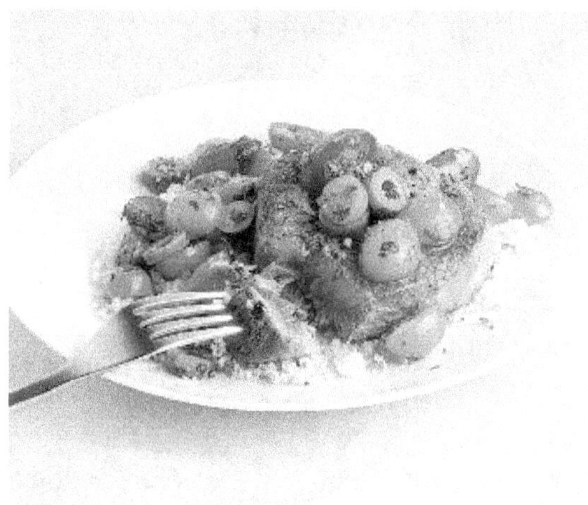

Tuna fillets with all tomatoes salad is a wonder food for bodybuilders and fitness lovers. Not only does tuna provide nutrients the body needs to maintain health, but those nutrients (protein, carbs and fat) are balanced in such a way that makes tuna idea for fitness and weight loss programs.

Canned tuna is also quick to prepare and is commonly eaten right out of the can or whipped into a tuna spread using fat-free mayonnaise with diced dill pickles which can be added to whole wheat sandwich bread or crackers, or used as a topping for salads. The only problem with canned tuna is that it can become a bit monotonous eating it the same way time after time.

Ingredients

- 4 tuna steaks without skin.

- 2 tablespoons of extra virgin olive oil.

- 1 shallot medium, finely chopped.

- 180 grs. Of yellow and red cherry tomatoes mixed, cut in half.

- 50 grs. Of green olives without bone, sliced.

- 2 tablespoons fresh basil, finely chopped.

- ½ tablespoon of lemon juice.

- Sea salt and freshly ground black pepper.

Preparation

Season the tuna steaks with one teaspoon of salt and ¼ tablespoon of pepper. Heat the oil in a large magefesa skillet over medium-high heat. Place the tuna in the pan in a single layer and cook, turning once, until it is made based on your preferences. Estimate about 3 or 4 minutes on average. Transfer the tuna to a large dish and reserve.

Reduce to medium heat and add the shallot to the pan. Cook, stirring, until golden brown, about 1 minute. Add the tomatoes, olives, basil, ½ teaspoon of salt, and a pinch of ground pepper. Cook until the tomatoes begin to acquire a smooth texture, about 2 minutes more. Remove the pan from the heat and slowly add the lemon juice. Pour the tomato salad over the reserved tuna steaks and serve.

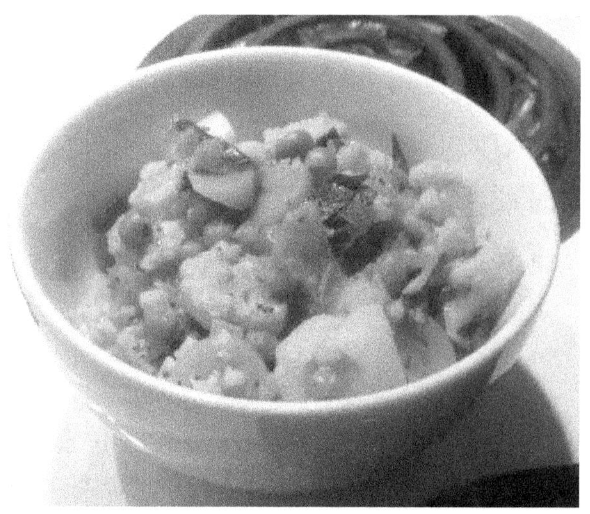

It's basically different vegetables cooked with spices and curry flavors, and when it's made well, it can be a great way to get tons of veggies into your diet. It's low in calories, high in fiber, and you don't even realize how much veggies you're eating because it is so flavorful!

Ingredients:

- ➢ 40 grams of cooked cauliflower
- ➢ 1 cup of frozen peas
- ➢ Three units of tomato
- ➢ Four units of ajetes
- ➢ One pinch of salt
- ➢ One pinch of ground black pepper
- ➢ One tablespoon dessert curry powder
- ➢ One carrot unit
- ➢ One handful of fresh cilantro
- ➢ 100 milliliters of water

> Three tablespoons of olive oil

Preparation

Gather all the ingredients to make the pea and tomato curry. This recipe is also very good with vegetables such as zucchini or broccoli.

Clean the young garlic by removing the green end and the lower part of the stems. Cut them as indicated in the image and sauté them in a pan with olive oil for a couple of minutes.

Peel the carrots, and then cut it into slices and add it to the pan. Let cook for 3 minutes.

Next, add the tomato peeled and cut into squares. Add a little salt and ground pepper, let cook for 5 minutes.

At this moment incorporate the curry. I have used a prepared mixture of spices for curry, similar to the great masala.

It is necessary that the curry is cooked with the rest of the ingredients for a couple of minutes over medium heat. After that time add the water and let it boil for another 3 minutes.

Add the frozen peas and get them to boil with the remaining ingredients for 2 minutes.

Finally, add the cooked cauliflower and let it mix well with the chickpea and tomato curry. The cauliflower makes the dish more consistent and gives us potassium and calcium.

Serve the vegan curry of peas and tomato with basmati rice or jasmine rice. If you are thinking of other recipes with curry you can try the green curry with prawns or the quinoa curry. Hope you like it.

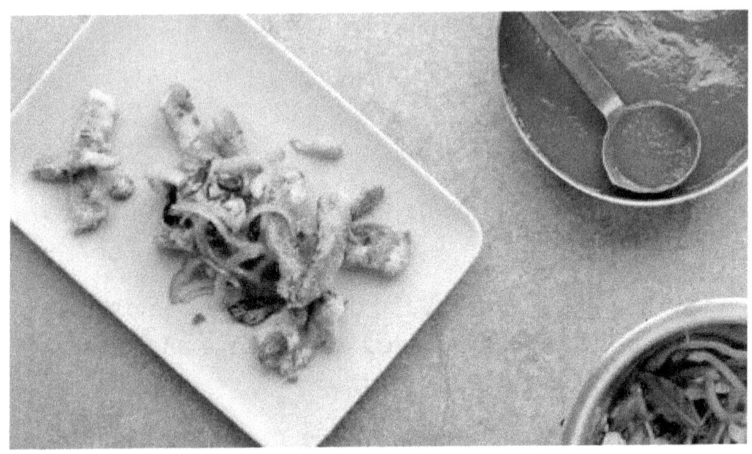

This recipe goes back to persian origins.

Makes 4 servings

It can be served cold or hot.

Ingredients

> - 4 slices of swordfish about ½ inch thick
>
> - Salt and pepper to taste
>
> - 1 cup of all-purpose flour
>
> - 1 teaspoon dried oregano
>
> - 1 teaspoon old bay seasoning
>
> - ¼ cup of vegetable oil

For pickling

> - 1 red pepper, without seeds or veins, cut into finite strips
>
> - 1 yellow pepper, without seeds or veins, cut into finite strips
>
> - 1 green pepper, without seeds or veins, cut into finite strips

> ➢ 1 medium red onion cut in julienne

➢ 2 garlic cloves, crushed

➢ ¼ cup of olive oil

➢ 1 teaspoon sweet paprika

➢ ½ cup of black olives, without seeds, cut into small pieces

➢ 1/3 cup capers

➢ 2 bay leaves

➢ ¾ cup of red vinegar

➢ 2 tablespoons of tomato paste

➢ 2 cups of fish stock

➢ Salt and pepper to taste

Preparation

1. Season the fish with salt and then pepper and sprinkle the flour, already mixed with oregano and old bay seasoning.

2. In little hot oil, brown the fish about 3 to 4 minutes per side, depending on the thickness of each piece — place in a glass baking dish.

3. Lightly cook the peppers, onions, and garlic in the hot olive oil, for about 3 to 4 minutes. Turn off the fire. Add the olives, capers, bay leaf and stir.

4. In a small saucepan, heat the red vinegar, tomato paste, and broth until it has been reduced by one third.

5. Add the mixture to the fish and then add the broth reduction. To make it taste better, let it marinate about 8 hours or overnight.

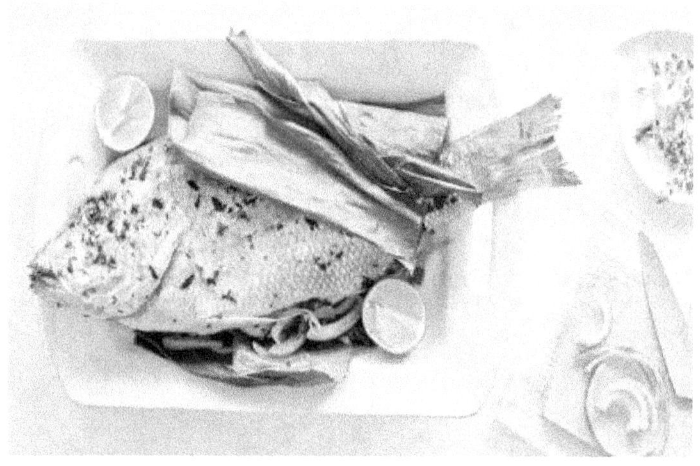

Snapper stuffed with vegetables in banana leaf

Makes 4 servings

Ingredients

- 4 complete, fresh, clean snappers (about 2 pounds each)

- Juice of 2 green lemons

- 1 spoonful of finely chopped fresh oregano leaves; reserve the twigs

- 1 tablespoon of finely chopped fresh thyme leaves; reserve the twigs

- 1 teaspoon sweet paprika

- 7 garlic cloves, 4 finely chopped, 3 very thin slices

- ⅓ cup of olive oil

- 1½ tablespoons of salt

- 2 tablespoons of sherry vinegar

- 1½ tablespoons of salt

- ➢ ¼ tablespoon of pepper

- ➢ Red onion, cut in slices

- ➢ 1 medium spanish onion, cut into slices

- ➢ 1 carrot, cut into thin slices

- ➢ 4 banana leaves

Preparation

1. Heat grill, already clean and oiled, over medium heat (350 ° f). Make incisions in the fish so that it absorbs the flavors better.

2. Cover the fish with the green lemon juice.

3. Mix the leaves of oregano, thyme, paprika, minced garlic, oil, salt and pepper, and vinegar. Place half of the marinade on the fish, cover with plastic wrap and let stand 30 minutes in the fridge.

4. Remove from the refrigerator and let it reach room temperature (about 20 minutes).

5. Cut 4 banana leaves to double the size of the fish. Cut 4 sheets of 12-inch square aluminum foil.

6. Put the banana leaves on the foil. Place one fish in each and fill with carrots, onions, slices of garlic, sprigs of thyme and oregano. Salt and pepper to taste (optional).

7. Pour the rest of the marinade divided among the fish. Cover well and put on direct heat for 20-25 minutes, depending on the thickness of the fish.

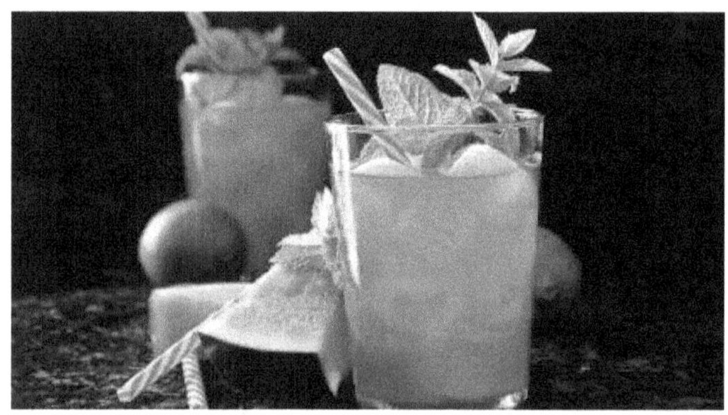

Use any melon you have on hand. You can also choose to use a rum flavored with melon.

Makes 1 a glass of 10 ounces.

Ingredients

- 6 to 10 fresh mint leaves, plus 1 sprig to decorate

- 1 small file, cut in half, plus a slice to decorate

- ¼ cup melon in pieces (use any type, such as cantaloupe, chinese melon or watermelon), plus some small pieces to garnish

- 2 tablespoons of simple stevia syrup or simple sugar syrup

- 1 line (1½ ounces) of white rum or rum flavored with melon

- 1 cup of ice

- ½ cup of soda water

Preparation

1. Place the mint leaves in a strong glass.

2. Squeeze the lime halves over the mint. Use a crusher to crush the mint and extract the aromatic oils lightly.

3. Add the melon and lightly squeeze it with the crusher.

4. Pour the syrup and rum into the glass, stirring. Stretch the preparation, if you prefer.

5. Add ice and soda water. Stir

6. Dress the glass with the sprig of mint, the slice of the lime and the small pieces of melon, and let the melon pieces float in the drink.

Chapter 7: Ways to Lose Stubborn Belly Fat

Belly fat is not just a problem because it can seem bad.

In fact, having a lot of fat in the abdominal area is closely related to diseases like type 2 diabetes and heart disease.

For this reason, belly fat loss is very beneficial to your health and can help you live longer.

Belly fat is usually estimated by measuring the circumference around your waist. This can easily be done at home with a simple tape measure.

A waistline too big is known as abdominal obesity for anything greater than 102 cm in men and 88 cm in women.

If you have a lot of fat around your waist, you should take some steps to get rid of it even if you are not very heavy.

Fortunately, there are some proven strategies for targeting fat in the belly area more than other areas of the body.

Here are 15ways based on evidence to lose belly fat.

1. Do not eat sugar and avoid sugary drinks

The added sugar is very unhealthy.

Studies show that it has unique harmful effects on metabolic health.

Sugar is half glucose, half fructose and fructose can only be metabolized by the liver in significant amounts.

When you eat a lot of added sugar, the liver is overloaded with fructose and is forced to turn it into fat.

Many studies have shown that an excess of sugar, mainly due to large amounts of fructose, can lead to increased accumulation of fat in the belly and liver.

Some think it is the main mechanism responsible for the harmful effects of sugar on health. It increases abdominal fat and liver fat, resulting in insulin resistance and a host of metabolic problems.

Liquid sugar is even worse in this regard. Liquid calories are not "saved" by the brain in the same way as solid calories. So when you drink sweet drinks, you end up eating more total calories.

Studies show that sugary drinks are associated with an increased risk of obesity of 60% in children, for each daily serving.

Make the decision to minimize the amount of sugar in your diet and consider completely eliminating sugary drinks.

This includes sweet sodas, fruit juices and various energy drinks with a high sugar content.

Remember that none of this applies to whole fruits, which are extremely healthy and contain a lot of fiber that mitigates the negative effects of fructose.

The amount of fructose you get from fruits is negligible compared to what you get from a diet high in refined sugar.

If you want to reduce refined sugar, you have to start reading the labels. Even foods marketed as health foods can contain large amounts of sugar.

2. Eating more protein is an excellent long-term strategy for reducing abdominal fat

Proteins are the most important macronutrient for losing weight.

It has been shown to reduce cravings by 60%, increase metabolism by 80 to 100 calories a day and help you consume up to 441 fewer calories a day.

If your goal is weight loss, adding protein may be the most effective change you can make to your diet.

Not only will this help you lose weight, but it will also help you avoid weight gain if you decide to give up your weight loss efforts.

There is also evidence that protein is particularly effective against belly fat.

One study showed that the amount and quality of protein consumed was inversely related to fat in the belly. In other words, people who ate more protein and better quality had a lot less abdominal fat.

Another study showed that the protein was linked to a significant reduction in the risk of abdominal fat gain over a 5-year period.

This study also showed that carbohydrates and refined oils were linked to an increase in the amount of fat in the belly, but that fruits and vegetables were linked to reduced amounts.

Many of the studies showing that proteins were effective contained protein at 25-30% of calories. That's what you should aim for.

Make an effort to increase your intake of protein - rich foods such as whole eggs, fish, seafood, legumes, nuts, meat and dairy products. These are the best sources of protein in the diet.

If you're struggling to get enough protein in your diet, a quality protein supplement (such as whey protein) is a healthy and convenient way to increase your total intake.

Additional tip: consider cooking your food in coconut oil. Some studies have shown that 30 ml (about 2 tablespoons) of coconut oil a day slightly reduces abdominal fat.

3. Cut the carbs out of your diet

Carbohydrate restriction is a very effective way to lose fat.

This is supported by many studies. When people reduce their carbohydrates, their appetite decreases and they lose weight.

More than 20 randomized controlled trials have now shown that low-carbohydrate diets lead to weight loss 2 to 3 times higher than low-fat diets.

This is true even when low-carbohydrate groups are allowed to eat as much as they wish, while low-fat groups have reduced caloric intake and are hungry.

Low carbohydrate diets also result in a rapid reduction in water weight, giving people almost instant results. A difference on the scale is often seen within 1-2 days.

There are also studies comparing low carb and fat diets, showing that low carb diets specifically target fat in the belly, organs and liver.

This means that a particularly high proportion of fat lost with a low carbohydrate diet is dangerous fat and conducive to abdominal diseases.

Avoiding refined carbohydrates (sugar, sweets, white bread, etc.) Should be enough, especially if you maintain a high protein intake.

However, if you need to lose weight fast, consider dropping your carbs at 50 grams a day. This will put your body into ketosis, killing your appetite and making your body start burning primarily fat as a source of energy.

Of course, low carb diets have many other health benefits in addition to weight loss. They can have life-saving effects in type 2 diabetics, for example.

4. Eat foods rich in fiber, especially viscous fiber

Dietary fiber is mainly non-digestible vegetable matter.

It is often said that eating a lot of fiber can help you lose weight.

This is true, but we must not forget that all the fibers are not equal.

It seems that it is mainly the soluble and viscous fibers that act on your weight.

These are fibers that bind water and form a thick gel that is found in the intestine.

This gel can significantly slow the flow of food in your digestive system and slow down the digestion and absorption of nutrients. The end result is a feeling of prolonged fullness and a loss of appetite.

One study found that 14 grams of extra fiber a day was linked to a 10% decrease in caloric intake and a 4.5 lb (2 kg) weight loss over 4 months.

In a five-year study, consumption of 10 grams of soluble fiber per day was associated with a 3.7% reduction in the amount of fat in the abdominal cavity.

This implies that soluble fiber can be particularly effective at reducing harmful abdominal fat.

The best way to get more fiber is to eat a lot of plant foods like vegetables and fruits. Legumes are also a good source, as are some cereals such as whole oats.

Then you can also try to take a fiber supplement such as glucomannan. It is one of the most viscous dietary fibers in existence and has been shown to cause weight loss in several studies.

5. Exercise is very effective at reducing belly fat

Exercise is important for a variety of reasons.

This is one of the best things you can do if you want to live long and healthy and avoid diseases.

The list of all the amazing benefits of exercise for health are beyond the scope of this guide, but exercise seems to be effective in reducing belly fat.

However, keep in mind that i am not talking about abdominal exercises here. The one-off reduction (fat loss in one place) is not possible, and doing endless exercises will not make you lose belly fat.

In one study, 6 weeks of training aimed only at the abdominal muscles had no measurable effect on waist circumference or the amount of fat in the abdominal cavity.

That said, other types of exercises can be very effective.

Aerobic exercise (such as walking, running, swimming, etc.) Has been shown to lead to significant reductions in abdominal fat in many studies.

Another study showed that exercise completely prevented people from regaining abdominal fat after losing weight, which implies that exercise is especially important when maintaining weight.

Exercise also reduces inflammation, lowers blood sugar, and improves all other metabolic abnormalities associated with excess abdominal fat.

6. Track your food and determine exactly what you eat and how much

What you eat is important. Almost everyone knows it.

However, most people do not have a clue what they actually eat.

People think they eat "high-protein", "low-carbohydrate" or whatever, but tend to overestimate or underestimate the number of calories they actually consume.

I think for anyone who really wants to optimize their diet, keeping track of their consumption for a while is absolutely essential and a vital step in a food program.

This does not mean you have to weigh everything up and measure for the rest of your life, but doing it from time to time for a few days at a time can help you understand where you need to make changes.

If you want to increase your protein intake to 25-30% of calories, as recommended above, it will not be enough to eat more protein-rich foods. You really need to measure and refine to achieve this goal.

Use a calorie calculator or a free online app to track what you eat.

I do it personally every few months. I weigh and measure everything i eat to see what my current diet looks like.

Then, i know exactly where to make adjustments to get closer to my goals.

7. Limit alcohol consumption

Alcohol is one of the first causes of fat accumulated in the stomach. In fact, in addition to stimulating the appetite, alcoholic beverages are very caloric. This is not indicated on the labels, but a glass of white wine contains about 100 calories and a 33cl beer about 125 calories. These calories are so-called "empty" calories since alcohol provides absolutely no nutrients to the body.

In addition, alcohol is responsible for slowing the elimination of fat. It is for this reason that it promotes the accumulation of fat on the stomach.

By reducing alcohol consumption and limiting it to exceptional occasions, abdominal fat will decrease quite rapidly.

8. Do cardio sport

To lose weight and fat, it is recommended to do at least 3 sports sessions a week, lasting between 30 and 45 minutes.

The so-called cardio sports are those that burn the most calories by stimulating the metabolism. They allow a noticeable and rapid loss of weight and fat. Running and cycling are some of the most effective cardio sports for losing abdominal fat, with skipping rope.

To further boost the combustion effect, the sport can be practiced on waking fasting. The body will then have to draw on its reserves during the effort and will directly attack the accumulated fat.

9. Monitor your diet closely

Abdominal fat is often linked to too much calorie intake. If the body ingests more calories than it spends, it will logically tend to store. To lose belly fat, you must ensure that its energy intake is not excessive. The nutritional recommendations are 2 400-2 600 calories per day for men and 1 800 to 2200 calories per day for women, depending on the size, weight and level of physical activity.

It is not enough to control the number of calories, it is also necessary to limit fatty and sweet foods such as sausages and pastries. Indeed, these foods are the most complicated to digest. A longer digestion time encourages the body to store, especially on the stomach.

To lose fat, you have to focus on protein and fiber on your plate. They are both digestible and satiating.

Care must be taken not to skip meals because the body stores when it is deprived.

10. Drink water and green tea

Drinking water regularly is important to regulate metabolism and help control appetite. Water also promotes the elimination of toxins and helps purify the body. On the other hand, the sparkling waters are to be avoided because the gas which they contain causes bloating.

Another important ally for losing belly fat is green tea. Green tea is diuretic: it helps to drain the body and fight against water retention. But green tea is also an excellent fat-burning thanks to the catechins it contains.

Several scientific studies have shown that catechins have the remarkable ability to stimulate fat oxidation and increase energy expenditure. People who consume green tea regularly accumulate less body fat and have a lower waistline than average.

To feel the benefits, you must consume at least 3 cups of green tea a day.

11. Make sure you have a good night's sleep

One in five people suffers from insomnia and sleep deficiency. But short nights of sleep promote weight gain and storage of fat, especially on the stomach.

Sleep is fundamental for the proper regulation of our metabolism. A short sleep time can undermine all efforts made elsewhere to lose abdominal fat.

In addition, beyond the physiological aspect, lack of sleep increases fatigue. It is scientifically proven that fatigue favors cravings, nibbling and craving for fatty and sugary foods.

According to the study "sleep and nutrition" of the national institute of sleep and vigilance conducted in 2015, the risk of obesity is increased by 50% in men and 34% in women short sleepers compared to long sleepers.

12. Remove the salt shaker from your table

Too much salt can make you swell.

Salt, in moderation, is a good thing - the mineral is necessary for the health of the heart and brain. But too much salt and you hold the water, swelling like a water balloon. Salt reduction is one of the main ways to reduce the weight of water (one of the reasons you can lose a lot of weight when you start a new diet!). Remove the salt shaker from your table so you do not have the habit of salting all your food. So if you taste your food and still want some salt, you can always get up and get it

13. Spit out your gum

Chewing gum causes bloating of the belly.

Many people chew gum to quell cravings or to avoid eating without thinking, but this tactic can have an unfortunate side effect: bloated stomach. Everyone naturally swallows a small amount of air when they chew, but it is magnified for people who chew gum, causing gas and bloating. In addition, it has been shown that some artificial sweeteners increase your appetite for junk food, so the gum could increase your waistline on two fronts.

14. Get to work in the bathroom

Constipation could be the culprit.

Nearly 20% of americans suffer from chronic constipation and permanent constipation can affect your entire body, including uncomfortable bloating and swelling of your stomach. Test constipation remedies that work for you so you do not have to suffer anymore.

15. Say no to processed foods

Processed foods contain a lot of salt.

Processed foods are one of the biggest sources of salt in the diet of americans and canadians, and what is frightening is that you probably do not even realize it. Because of the way these addictive foods are formulated, salt is hidden in all sorts of things, from soups to pasta sauces, even so it's the same for sweet cakes in a box. Swap processed foods for fresh food and your belly will thank you for it. Not only will you lose salt swelling, you will also lose extra empty calories and lose weight.

7-day flat-belly meal plan

Follow this menu "flat stomach in 7 days" to lose inches of waist.

Getting rid of belly fat is not limited to skinny jeans: research shows that people with less visceral fat (the fat that surrounds your organs and that gives an impression of swollen belly) have a reduced risk of diabetes-type 2 and heart disease.

So, not only will fat loss help you feel better, but it will also help prevent some health problems.

Although there is not one magic food that melt belly fat, studies have reported that some foods have special benefits such as:

- Avocado,

- Artichokes,

- Whole grains,

- Kefir,

- Green tea,

- Eggs,

- The peanuts

- And chickpeas.

These foods work in different ways to help reduce fat cells and reduce waist circumference.

This 7-day meal plan incorporates these "flat stomach" foods, with vegetables, whole grains, fruits, healthy fats and proteins, to help with the loss of belly fat.

Lose weight: day 1

Flat belly bonus: chickpeas are "flat stomach" foods with 5 grams of fiber and 5 grams of protein per 100 grams. These nutrients fill you up and stabilize your blood sugar to keep you filled.

In addition, chickpea eaters generally have waistlines that are less than 5 centimeters tall for those who do not eat them.

Breakfast (about 342 calories and 4 g of fiber)

- Half a medium avocado and a quarter kale

- 230 ml of green tea

Pre-lunch snacks (about 182 calories and 5 grams of fiber)

Cucumber salad:

- 225 grams of cucumber slices

- 1 c. Lemon juice

- 1 pinch of salt and pepper

- Dried dill for taste (optional)

Mix the cucumber slices, lemon juice, salt, pepper and dill in a bowl for a quick and easy cucumber salad.

- 8 whole wheat crackers

Lunch (about 388 calories and 8 grams of fiber)

Chickpea salad:

- 1 c. Olive oil and red wine vinegar

- 2 tablespoons chopped parsley

- 150 grams of salad (any)

- 1/2 bowl of grated carrots

- 60 grams of broccoli florets, roughly chopped

- 55 grams of chickpeas,

- 3 c. Chopped red onion

- 2 tablespoons crumbled feta cheese

Mix the olive oil, vinegar and parsley to make the vinaigrette. Combine green vegetables, carrots, broccoli, chickpeas, onion and cheese in a bowl. Mix with the vinaigrette.

The snack (about 111 calories and 2 g of fiber):

- 2 tablespoons spicy peanuts

Dinner (about 488 calories and 16 grams of fiber)

- 2 bowls of vegetable soup. The recipe

- 1 c. Olive oil, balsamic vinegar and dijon mustard

- 1/2 c. Dried oregano

- 150 grams of salad (any)

Whisk together the oil, vinegar, mustard and oregano. Then mix the salad with the vinaigrette.

- 1 round of 4-inch whole wheat pita

- 60 grams of hummus

Keep what's left for the next day.

Daily totals: *1,511 calories, 50 g protein, 134 g carbohydrate, 35 g fiber, 92 g fat, 2,205 mg sodium*

Lose weight: day 2

Flat stomach bonus: research has shown that eating nuts is associated with a thinner waistline and a lower bmi.

In addition, spicy peanuts can help boost your metabolism with capsaicin.

Breakfast (about 309 calories and 12 g of fiber)

Muesli with kefir and berries:

- 120 ml of kefir

- 40 grams of unsweetened muesli

- 65 grams of raspberries

Beside:

- 230 ml of green tea

Pre-lunch snacks (about 95 calories and 4 g of fiber)

- 1 medium-sized apple

Lunch: (about 384 calories and 12 g of fiber)

- 2 bowls of vegetable soup.

- 1 round of 4-inch whole wheat pita, grilled

- 60 grams of hummus

The snack (about 166 calories and 3 g of fiber)

- 3 tablespoons spicy peanuts

Dinner (about 521 calories and 11 g of fiber)

- 140 grams of oriental chickpeas.

- 1 c. Olive oil, balsamic vinegar and dijon mustard

- 150 grams of salad (any)

Whisk together the oil, vinegar and mustard. Mix the salad with the vinaigrette.

Daily totals: *1475 calories, 48 grams of protein, 178 grams of carbohydrates, 42 grams of fiber, 75 grams of fat, 1,402 mg of sodium*

Lose weight: day 3

Flat belly bonus: green tea contains compounds called catechins that can protect against obesity. In addition, caffeine slightly increases your metabolism.

Breakfast (about 306 calories and 9 g of fiber)

- 480 ml of red berry kefir smoothie

- 230 ml of green tea

Pre-lunch snacks (about 223 calories and 4 g of fiber)

- 6 whole wheat crackers

- 1 tablespoon peanut butter

Lunch (about 335 calories and 8 g of fiber)

- 1 vegetarian wrap and a half.

The snack (about 105 calories and 3 g of fiber)

- 1 medium sized banana

Dinner (about 517 calories and 7 g of fiber)

- 100 grams of salmon steak with honey and orange sauce.

- 2 rings of apple "donuts" to taste for dessert. For this you will need, 1 medium apple, 3 tablespoons of almond butter and 2 teaspoons of unsweetened grated coconut.

Note: cook extra quinoa for other days of the week.

Daily totals: *1,496 calories, 69 grams of protein, 188 grams of carbohydrates, 30 grams of fiber, 59 grams of fat, 1,251 mg of sodium*

Lose weight: day 4

Flat belly bonus: high-fiber lenses nourish healthy intestinal bacteria and promote fluidity of the bowel to prevent bloating and constipation.

Adding dark green leafy vegetables (as we do in tonight's dinner) helps you take fewer calories without increasing hunger.

According to research from harvard university, vegetables are the number one food that promotes weight loss.

Breakfast (about 338 calories and 8 grams of fiber)

- 350 ml of green tea
- 1 toast to the avocado.
- 2 kiwis

Pre-lunch snacks (about 139 calories and 3 grams of fiber)

- 1 hard-boiled egg seasoned with a pinch of salt and pepper
- 1 medium orange

Lunch (about 379 calories and 13 g of fiber)

- Chickpea salad.

The snack (about 166 calories and 3 g of fiber)

- 3 c. Spicy peanuts

Dinner (about 453 calories and 14 g of fiber)

- 80 grams of vegetables, salad and lentils.

Daily totals: 1475 calories, 63 grams of protein, 177 grams of carbohydrates, 41 grams of fiber, 65 grams of fat, 1709 mg of sodium

Lose weight: day 5

Flat belly bonus: whole grains (such as quinoa and brown rice) help to lose weight.

Breakfast (about 309 calories and 12 g of fiber)

Muesli with kefir and berries

- 120 ml of kefir

- 45 grams of unsweetened muesli

- 125 g raspberries

Beside :

- 230 ml green tea

Pre-lunch snacks (about 247 calories and 7 grams of fiber)

- 6 whole wheat crackers

- 1 medium carrot, cut into sticks

- 60 grams of hummus

Lunch (about 351 calories and 9 g of fiber)

- 100 grams of quinoa salad with roasted vegetables, chickpea and cherry tomatoes.

Taste (about 95 calories and 4 g of fiber)

- 1 medium-sized apple

Dinner (about 497 calories and 8 g of fiber)

- 80 grams of zucchini spaghetti with avocado pesto.

Daily totals: *1,498 calories, 63 grams of protein, 180 grams of carbohydrates, 42 grams of fiber, 68 grams of fat, 1,455 mg of sodium*

Lose weight: day 6

Flat belly bonus: people who regularly eat avocado are more likely to have a smaller size. It's true that avocados are high in fat, but it's the right guy who keeps your heart healthy and fills you up.

Breakfast (about 338 calories and 8 grams of fiber)

- 350 ml of green tea

- 1 toast with avocado

- 2 kiwis

Pre-lunch snacks (about 78 calories and 0 g of fiber)

- 1 hard-boiled egg seasoned with a pinch of salt and pepper

Lunch (about 360 calories and 13 g of fiber)

- White bean salad with vegetables and balsamic vinaigrette.

Pre-lunch, snacks: (about 223 calories and 4 g of fiber)

- 6 whole wheat crackers

- 1 tablespoon peanut butter

Dinner (about 483 calories and 11 g of fiber)

- 75 grams of shrimp

- 80 grams of sauteed spinach.

- 150 grams of cooked whole wheat orzo

- 1 c. Tablespoon of olive oil

- 2 tbsp. Chopped fresh parsley

Mix the orzo with the oil and parsley.

Daily totals: *1,483 calories, 78 grams of protein, 144 grams of carbohydrates, 37 grams of fiber, 71 grams of fat, 1,689 mg of sodium*

Lose weight: day 7

Flat belly bonus: protein from eggs can help you lose weight and build muscle. Eat quality protein at meals throughout the day.

Breakfast (about 307 calories and 5 g of fiber)

Scrambled eggs with spicy sauce

- 2 eggs, scrambled

- 1 tablespoon of hot sauce

- 1 tablespoon crumbled cheese

- 1 tablespoon chopped fresh cilantro

- A pinch of crushed red pepper (optional)

- 1 slice of whole wheat bread, toasted

Beside :

- 1 medium orange

- 230 ml green tea

Pre-lunch snacks (about 210 calories and 5 g of fiber)

- 1 tablespoon peanut butter

- 1 c. Hot water, more if needed

- 1 medium banana, sliced

Mix the peanut butter and water to make a sauce to sprinkle on the banana slices.

Lunch (about 362 calories and 17 grams of fiber)

- 2 toasts with avocado and white beans.

- 1 c. Tablespoon of olive oil

- 2 tbsp. Balsamic vinegar

- 1 c. Dijon mustard

- 1/2 c. Dried oregano

- 150 grams of salad (any)

Whisk together the oil, vinegar and mustard. Mix the salad with the vinaigrette.

- 40 grams of raspberries

The snack (about 123 calories and 3 g of fiber)

Cucumber salad:

- 225 grams of cucumber slices

- 1 c. Lemon juice

- A pinch of salt and pepper

- Dried dill (optional)

Mix the cucumber slices, lemon juice, salt, pepper and dill in a bowl for a quick and easy cucumber salad.

- 5 whole wheat crackers

Dinner (about 504 calories and 11 g of fiber)

- 80 grams of hasselback chicken.

- 100 grams of cooked whole wheat orzo

- 1/2 c. Dried oregano

Daily totals: 1,507 calories, 82 grams of protein, 161 grams of carbohydrates, 41 grams of fiber, 66 grams of fat, 1,920 mg of sodium

One of the commonly asked questions about intermittent fasting is usually "won't i get hungry? As mentioned above, the fact that you're not hungry is all about the pattern your body is used to. If you eat something during the day, or if you have a particular hour you eat every day, your body will get used to this order and start preparing insulin for food. However, after a short period of acclimatization, your body will also accept a new order.

Remember, your body's physical and cognitive abilities are not adversely affected by fasting.

Where do i receive the energy to do sports? Will, i do not get tired if i am hungry, or will i be able to complete my workouts? After your body becomes used to the unique order, even if you don't eat before sports, it starts working as usual.

Even training on empty stomach results in better metabolic adaptation, i.e. Better performance, increased muscle protein synthesis, and a greater anabolic response to post-sport food; in other words, when you do sports when you eat both you eat, and you will earn the muscles you deserve.

When doing sports, you can arrange your open window to fit your sports schedule. The crucial thing here is that if you are not an athlete who needs to perform at any moment, you should not worry and don't panic. If you only want to lose a few pounds or muscle, try to do your best.

Can fasting cause muscle loss? This is one of the most asked questions in the mind of people who want to apply intermittent fasting. But it's a baseless concern. Because "the body's hourly protein amount of 30 grams for several hours if you do not take your body begins to use your muscles as a source of energy" is not true information.

A study shows that the body protects muscles even in the event of hunger. In other words, the body's process of protein processing can take longer than said. On the other hand, spreading the total amount of protein you need to take all day or consuming in a short time does not make any difference to your body.

So if i don't eat for a long time, will my body go through starvation?". The thought process here is as follows: since our body thinks that we cannot get the necessary calories when we do not eat, we begin to store the limited calories you take instead of burning; therefore, the weight loss effect of starvation disappears. However, this approach is not entirely correct, either. Martin, one of the authors of lean gain, clarifies:

- ❖ 60 the earliest time the body recognizes hunger and lowers metabolic rate is 60 hours. According to different studies, the metabolic rate is not affected by fasting before 72-96 hours.

- ❖ On the other hand, although it may seem like a paradox, the metabolic rate rises in short-term hunger situations. To give clear figures, research has reported an increase of 3.6% to 10% in 36-48 hours of fasting.

- ❖ Epinephrine and norepinephrine (adrenaline and noradrenaline) sharpen the mind and make us active. Behavior like hunting and hunting increases the chances of survival. At some point, for example, if you don't eat for a few days, it's more advantageous if the body stores what you eat."

If your diet provides you with benefits such as muscle development, weight loss, reduction in body fat, and you are healthy, continue using the same method. However, if what you're doing isn't working, you don't get the results you want, or it makes you feel bad, you can give it a different way. Trying something new is the most effective way to know if it will do you any good.

There are also contradictory ideas, such as those who argue that intermittent fasting diet practices have positive effects on health. The basis of these considerations is a number of studies showing that skipping breakfast meals increases the risk of cardiovascular disease. It should also be kept in mind that hunger lasting longer than 12 hours may increase the problems associated with gallbladder by 50%. And the latest endocrinology specialists' results in studies that increase the risk of diabetes, the amount of fat in the abdomen and not the fat, hints that applying it for long periods of time will not produce very safe results.

Conclusion

Should intermittent fasting diets be applied?

Fasting may be a dietary option that can be preferred as short-term administration in obese individuals who do not comply with daily calorie restriction. However, even if slimming begins in a short time, it should be kept in mind that intermittent fasting diets, such as fasting, may cause adverse side effects such as excessive hunger, headache and drop in blood sugar. Today, scientific data shows that long-term application can also pose risks that can cause more harm to health. For this reason, it can be provided to gain motivation towards a little slimming by applying in a short time. However, it should be noted that; the main rule that protects health and ensures healthy lasting is not hunger, but rather a variety of natural, consisting of 3 main and 1 intermediate meals, which are balanced from all nutrients that protect the body's health.

9 781695 868328